Praise for *TRICARE Around the World* by *J.D. Letaw*

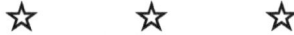

☆   ☆   ☆

"Indispensable resource for military families, retirees, and avid travelers . . . Answers the most pressing questions about obtaining medical care while overseas or when traveling across the USA. A must-read for any member of the military community."

Stephanie Montague, chief editor of
Poppin' Smoke military travel blog

"Simplifies TRICARE for <u>everyone</u> (all military families, not just expat ones) . . . The claims checklist alone is well worth the price of the book."

Doug Nordman, author of *The Military Guide to Financial Independence and Retirement*

"Even the TRICARE site is not organized this well. Gives detailed step-by-step procedures and many times also explains why they are so critical to follow."

Robert R. Crawford, Amazon reviewer

"I worked for the TRICARE program for 20 years, and I would highly recommend this book to all TRICARE beneficiaries."

Mikahela, Amazon reviewer

"As a recently retired US Army Reservist Family Practice physician, I have been asked by patients how to best use TRICARE. This book serves to demystify the process. The detailed instructions on how TRICARE works . . . and potential pitfalls make this book worth its price many times over . . . Understandable for those new to using TRICARE. For retired military members, this book is a must."

Robert S., TRICARE beneficiary and physician

"Excellent information in one place . . . gives you the confidence to make it all work."

Rob141, USAF (retired), Amazon reviewer

All information is believed to be accurate at the time of publishing. For inquiries or corrections, contact John@theTRICAREguy.com.

This book is available at bulk discount for non-profits, promotions, or premiums. Special editions, including tailored covers with corporate imprints, can be created for bulk purchase.

Editor: Jennifer L. Jansons
Cover art: Andrea Schmidt *(www.a-schmidt.com)*

ISBN: Paperback: 978-1-965461-02-0
        Kindle E-book: 978-1-965461-01-3

Publisher's Cataloging-in-Publication Data
Names: Letaw, John D., 1958- , author.
Title: The ultimate guide to TRICARE : getting the most from your
    military medical benefits/ J.D. Letaw.
Description: Honolulu, HI : Deep Blue C, 2025. | Summary: Covers all
    TRICARE plans for all beneficiaries (active duty, retirees,
    reservists, former spouses, etc.), including plan options, how to
    enroll, cost & benefits, and how to use worldwide. Detailed topics
    include filing claims, using TRICARE with VA healthcare, appeals,
    Medicare/Medicaid and options for special needs children.
Identifiers: LCCN: 2025905894 | ISBN 9781965461020 (pbk.) | ISBN
    9781965461013 (Kindle ebook)
Subjects: LCSH: Managed care plans (Medical care) – United States –
    Handbooks, manuals, etc. | United States. Office of the
    Assistant Secretary of Defense (Health Affairs). TRICARE
    Management Activity – Handbooks, manuals, etc. | United
    States – Armed Forces – Medical care – Handbooks, manuals,
    etc. | Travel – Health aspects. | LCGFT: Handbooks and
    manuals. | BISAC: MEDICAL / General. | MEDICAL / Reference.
Classification: RA413.5.U5 L48 2025 (print) | LCC RA413.5.U5
    (ebook) | DDC 362.1042580973--dc23
LC record available at https://lccn.loc.gov/2025905894

The Ultimate Guide to TRICARE®:

Getting the Most From Your
Military Medical Benefits

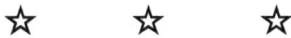

☆   ☆   ☆

J. D. LETAW

Deep Blue C Press
Honolulu, Hawaii

Table of Contents

Disclaimer

THIS PUBLICATION IS NOT SPONSORED, reviewed, or endorsed by any government agency. The author is not and never has been an employee or representative of TRICARE, Military Health System, or any TRICARE contractor.

Military medical benefits and costs are subject to change at any time, often with little notice. This can happen through legislation or by issuance of rules by appropriate authority. Information herein is believed to be accurate at the time of publication. Changes in pricing, benefits, or eligibility may have occurred since publication and may not be reflected in this book.

This book is not intended to be, and should not be construed as, medical advice or a definitive statement or commitment of benefits. The reader should verify critical information with their TRICARE provider or regional contractor. The author assumes no liability for inaccurate, incomplete, or outdated information in this book, nor for any inferences or conclusions that might be drawn from it.

Author's Note: Acronyms

ANYONE WHO HAS BEEN AROUND the military for any length of time knows that military speech is full of jargon and acronyms. This can be overwhelming to the newcomer because it seems like everyone around you is speaking a foreign language. We are sensitive to this throughout the book, and we believe that a large part of our mission is to educate our audience so that we can all participate more fully in discussions about health care.

As an aid to our readers, **Appendix B at the back of the book has a complete list of acronyms.** Refer to it often.

1
Getting Started

THIS BOOK IS THE RESULT OF DECADES OF EXPERIENCE traveling, living in the United States and overseas, and using different TRICARE® plans both as an active duty family and in retirement. We are privileged to lead a vibrant online community of more than 25,000 TRICARE users, giving us unmatched perspective of TRICARE in virtually every possible circumstance. This unprecedented global view, based on thousands of members' stories, reveals how TRICARE works around the world – not just our own first-person experience or reflecting the TRICARE "official" view – but what *really* happens, as we explain how to navigate your benefits with maximum effectiveness.

The first edition of this book, entitled *TRICARE Around the World*, was written in Thailand during the COVID lockdown in 2020. We were enrolled in Select as a retiree family and honed our skills by filing claims for all types of care overseas. The second edition was written in Hawaii, post-pandemic. Our family enrolled in Select rather than Prime even though we had a military hospital nearby. We will clarify in the book why we made this choice. Now that I am on Medicare and TRICARE for Life (TFL), this book provides greater detail about that transition and how to use TFL internationally. Our global experience, plus the stories of thousands of families like yours, offers a broad perspective on TRICARE usage worldwide.

TRICARE: A Life Skill

Despite how it might appear, TRICARE is not governed by mysterious forces of nature. There are specific rules and processes that you can learn and apply. Mastering your use of TRICARE is a skill that requires focus and intentionality. You would not teach yourself to swim by recklessly jumping into the deep end of a pool; likewise, **you do not want your first experience with your health plan to be in the midst of a crisis.** It is far better to start with small steps, so you'll be ready to face greater medical issues when they inevitably arise. This means using TRICARE for routine matters and filing simple claims at first so that you'll be prepared to handle medical emergencies later on. Train yourself so that you will be ready for whatever the future brings.

We run a number of Facebook groups where we interact daily with thousands of TRICARE beneficiaries[1]. Some of their stories are very uplifting; others are gut-wrenching. Quite routinely we encounter a frantic post that goes something like this:

> "Help! I just joined this group. We are in *(Spain, Korea, Reno, Nevada)*. My *(wife, husband, child)* just *(crashed a motorbike, got diagnosed with cancer, needs expensive medication)* and we don't know what to do. Do we need to go to a military hospital? Will TRICARE pay? How do we find an approved doctor? We're in a panic! Who do we call?"

This semi-fictitious post is an aggregation of actual requests within our online forum. Can you imagine a loved one suddenly becoming sick or injured in a country where you may not speak the language, don't understand the healthcare system, and are unsure what your health plan covers or how to use it? What if _you_ are incapacitated, and your spouse must figure this out on their own? What would they do?

Finding yourself in this situation is both tragic and unnecessary. The last thing you want to be doing in a crisis is scanning the internet, trying to figure out who to ask for help. In that moment, you need to be focused on your loved one, confidently guiding their care because you know what TRICARE

---

[1] You can find our Facebook groups, YouTube channel, and other resources by visiting our website at www.theTRICAREguy.com

will cover and how to use it. Facebook groups are **reactive** in nature: Someone posts a problem, and we help them through it. This book and our other resources are **proactive,** to educate you and your family **before** a crisis occurs. Obtaining this book is a huge first step. Keep reading and we'll walk you through each step of the process.

What is TRICARE?

TRICARE is a health program administered by the Defense Health Agency (DHA) and is part of the U.S. Military Health System (MHS). It is intended primarily for members of the uniformed services, retirees, medical retirees, certain Guard and Reservists, and their eligible family members. All TRICARE plans offer comprehensive coverage including preventive and wellness care, mental health care, pharmacy benefits, and a broad range of diagnostic and treatment services. Beneficiaries can get care either at a Military Treatment Facility (MTF) on base, or through civilian health care providers. TRICARE is NOT affiliated with the VA (Veterans Administration), and in general does not extend benefits to non-retired veterans.

TRICARE works basically the same whether in the United States or abroad. A notable exception is the Philippines, which has unique rules which are explained in Chapter 9. Despite the consistency of TRICARE worldwide, many beneficiaries find it challenging to use internationally for a variety of reasons:

- Network providers overseas are scarce, which means users commonly see non-network providers and must learn to file claims.

- International healthcare providers are less familiar with TRICARE and may not know how to validate your benefits or document your care.

- TRICARE users living or traveling abroad are often uncertain about which providers they are allowed to see.

The Ultimate Guide to TRICARE

- Healthcare norms and practices vary from country to country and can be baffling to Americans abroad.
- Language or cultural barriers can lead to further obstacles when seeking care outside the U.S.

This book will explain the usage of TRICARE both within the United States and in foreign countries.

Regions, Programs and Contractors

Different contractors manage the various TRICARE regions and programs. It is important to enroll in the right region so you will have easier access to your benefits. The contractors, regions and programs are:

- **Region: TRICARE East**
  - o Contractor: Humana Government Business
  - o www.tricare-east.com
  - o Includes Alabama, Connecticut, Delaware, Florida, Georgia, Indiana, Iowa (Rock Island Arsenal area only), Kentucky, Maine, Maryland, Massachusetts, Michigan, Mississippi, Missouri (St. Louis area only), New Hampshire, New Jersey, New York, North Carolina, Ohio, Pennsylvania, Rhode Island, South Carolina, Tennessee, Vermont, Virginia, Washington DC, and West Virginia.

- **Region: TRICARE West**
  - o Contractor: TriWest Healthcare Alliance (TriWest)
  - o tricare-bene.triwest.com
  - o Includes Alaska, Arizona, Arkansas, California, Colorado, Hawaii, Idaho, Illinois, Iowa (excluding Rock Island Arsenal area), Kansas, Louisiana, Minnesota, Missouri (excluding the St. Louis area), Montana, Nebraska, Nevada, New Mexico, North Dakota, Oklahoma, Oregon, South Dakota, Texas, Utah, Washington, Wisconsin, and Wyoming.

- **Region: TRICARE Overseas**
  - Contractor: International SOS (ISOS)
  - www.tricare-overseas.com
  - U.S. territories and all international locations

- **TRICARE for Life (TFL)**
  - Contractor: Wisconsin Physician Services (WPS)
  - www.tricare4u.com

- **U.S. Family Health Plan (USFHP)**
  - Various regional plans within the United States
  - www.usfhp.com

- **Express Scripts**
  - TRICARE pharmacy provider for retail, home delivery, and MTF prescriptions
  - militaryrx.express-scripts.com

- **Active Duty Dental Program (ADDP)/ TRICARE Dental Program (TDP)**
  - Contractor: United Concordia
  - ADDP: secure.addp-ucci.com
  - TDP: www.uccitdp.com

- **FEDVIP Vision and Dental Plans**
  - Optional fee-based vision and dental care for retirees, reservists, and eligible family members.
  - Run by the Office of Personnel Management (OPM)
  - Various plans offered by approved contractors
  - www.benefeds.com

Beware of confusion! TriWest is the contractor for both the TRICARE West Region and for VA Community Care Regions 4 and 5. If providers are not careful, bills might be sent to the wrong entity: TRICARE West instead of VA West, or vice versa. Both are managed by TriWest. If the bill is sent to the wrong processor, it would be rejected, leaving the patient to sort out the mess. **Do NOT say "TriWest"** at your doctor's office – **you must specify whether VA or TRICARE West will be paying, and make sure your provider is equally clear.**

To manage your health benefits online, use the website of your respective contractor. You will create an account to track claims, manage enrollment, and communicate about your benefits. You can have accounts for as many regions as you like without impacting your benefits. **If you anticipate international travel, we strongly encourage you to create an account on the TRICARE Overseas (TOS) site.** Creating an online account does not change your enrollment, but it will speed up any claims you might have for care while traveling internationally. It can be difficult or impossible to create a TOS web account while outside the USA, so do this before heading abroad.

The official TRICARE website at **tricare.mil** has a great deal of useful information, but **you will <u>not</u> have a log-in account or manage your care there.** The site provides a number of useful tools. Visit **The TRICARE Guy YouTube channel** for demonstration and explanation of these tools. You also can read about this in Chapter 14.

If you travel back-and-forth between regions, you do not need to switch plans or regions as you travel. Simply choose the region in which you spend the most time and enroll there. Mobile families will find it advantageous to be in Select for reasons that will be explained later. Regardless of which plan or region in which you are enrolled, you are always able to seek emergency or urgent care without referral or pre-authorization. Chapter 5 explains how to find providers in a variety of situations.

When you become eligible for Medicare, you must enroll in Medicare Parts A and B to maintain your TRICARE benefits, even if you live overseas. Part A is free, but there is a fee for Part B. Enrolling in Medicare Part B automatically places you in TRICARE for Life (TFL), which can be used worldwide. All of this is explained in Chapter 8, along with certain exceptions to enrollment deadlines.

Group A vs. Group B

In 2018, a two-tiered pricing structure was introduced. Members will fall into one of two groups.

- **Group A** consists of members whose initial date of service is prior to January 1, 2018. These members and their dependents were grandfathered into an earlier pricing structure.

- **Group B** consists of members and their dependents whose initial military service is on or after January 1, 2018. Other than active duty service members – for whom care is nearly always free – Group B members follow a newer pricing structure.

You will need to know which group you are in when reviewing your health care costs in Chapter 6. Call your regional contractor if you are unsure.

2021 Fee for TRICARE Select

On January 1, 2021, a **new enrollment fee** was initiated for many Group A retirees in TRICARE Select. Sponsors who are medically retired and their family members and survivors are exempt. Affected members were advised to arrange payment of this fee. **Those who failed to do this were eventually disenrolled from their TRICARE plan** and placed into a status of Direct Care Only (DCO). DCO is explained in Chapter 7; it provides access to primary care at an MTF **if** they can accommodate you. Care by civilian providers is not covered. You do NOT want to be in a DCO status.

If you are a Group A retiree in Select and have not used TRICARE since early 2021, **it is possible that you are no**

longer enrolled in a plan. Call your regional contractor to determine your status and see what alternatives are available to restore benefits for yourself and your family members.

2025 Realignment

On January 1, 2025, TriWest took over as regional contractor for the TRICARE West region. Concurrently, six states shifted from the East region to the West: Arkansas, Illinois, Louisiana, Oklahoma, Texas, and Wisconsin. Regrettably, this transition did not go smoothly; providers and families have faced a myriad of problems with claims, referrals, and payments.

Beneficiaries in the West region, including the six states listed above, were required to reestablish payment of their monthly fee if they are paying by credit card or bank transfer. It is likely that some members failed to do so. **If not rectified, they eventually will be disenrolled from their plan**. If you are in the West Region and have not used your TRICARE benefits since January 2025, please double check that your payments are set up and that all family members are enrolled in a plan to avoid complication when you seek care.

The extreme problems encountered during this transition may have led some families to walk away from their TRICARE plan. As of this writing, the issues are still ongoing, with slow resolution. Once these problems are resolved, we hope you will give TRICARE another chance. We continue to track and report on these issues in our Facebook group.

VA vs. TRICARE

A great many retired veterans also have VA benefits in addition to their TRICARE health plan. It is possible to use both TRICARE and VA, but your care must be coordinated to ensure everything is billed properly. We have compiled a number of tips for those in this situation. Please read Chapter 10 for an overview of using VA healthcare in conjunction with TRICARE.

Other Health Insurance (OHI)

Broadly speaking, health insurance policies come in one of two forms:

- Comprehensive health plans covering a broad range of health services or
- Medical supplements.

Comprehensive plans cover pretty much all your health needs. TRICARE refers to these policies as Other Health Insurance (OHI). By contrast, supplements cover only TRICARE copayments and deductibles and are _not_ considered to be OHI. Supplements and travel insurance are discussed later in this chapter.

Examples of OHI include:

- Employer-sponsored health plans
- Travel insurance that provides medical coverage
- National health plans when living abroad
- Policies purchased on the open market
- In 2024, TRICARE Overseas started referring to the VA Foreign Medical Program (FMP) as OHI, which has implications for disabled retirees living abroad. See Chapter 10 for a discussion of this.

By law, OHI is first payer: you _must_ claim your medical expenses on that policy first. Only after the OHI settles can remaining expenses be filed with TRICARE. **The exception to this is Medicaid,** with which TRICARE remains first payer. The rules governing the use of OHI are discussed in Chapter 13 ("When to File") and Appendix D. We generally find the purchase of OHI to be unnecessary and duplicative, making it harder to use your TRICARE benefits, but there are situations where it might make sense.

Buying another policy is a deeply personal decision that only you and your spouse can make. It goes beyond financial considerations. Some people lack confidence that TRICARE will be there when they need it, or perhaps they think it's too confusing. They may not be aware of the vast array of benefits available under TRICARE, or they buy an employer plan as the path of least resistance, not realizing this demotes TRICARE to a second-payer position. This lack of awareness needlessly costs families thousands of dollars each year.

In our view, the question is not whether TRICARE is too confusing. The real question is: ***Are you willing to expend the effort to learn how to use the benefits that you have earned through your service and sacrifice?*** Our view is that TRICARE is not hard to use; it is only hard to <u>learn</u> to use because, until now, there has been no comprehensive training. With the right learning tool, TRICARE is actually quite simple – and this book is that tool!

A financial comparison of TRICARE vs. a commercial plan might look something like this. These examples are broad generalizations and do not reflect any actual policy.

Annual premium
- TRICARE: $0-$4,000 per family (free for AD; higher costs for certain reservists)
- Commercial policy: $4,000-$10,000 per person,

Annual deductible
- TRICARE: $0-$700 per family
- Commercial policy: $2,000-$10,000 per family

Annual cap of out-of-pocket expenses
- TRICARE: $1000 - $5,000 maximum per family
- Commercial policy: $12,000+

A family could easily save $10,000 per year simply by rejecting employer-provided health coverage and using TRICARE instead. Doing this consistently for 20 years equates to

$200,000 in cost savings. Invest the savings to boost your nest egg and enhance your retirement!

Notify your regional contractor when you have OHI and when you cancel it. TRICARE claims will be rejected if you do not show proof that you have already filed with OHI first and received your final statement, known as an Explanation of Benefits (EOB). This is requested on DD Form 2642 (TRICARE claim form) and is taken quite seriously by TRICARE. Once your OHI policy has paid out, you can submit a TRICARE claim for any remaining unpaid balance. If your regional contractor erroneously thinks that you have OHI (perhaps because you did not notify them of cancellation), they will reject *all* your claims, thinking that you have not yet filed with your other policy. This issue comes up all the time in our Facebook group.

This matter of first payer/second payer is a big reason why I have never purchased any other insurance for my family. It's bad enough dealing with one insurer; why would I want to deal with two? I don't want two insurers bickering with each other. TRICARE has always taken good care of my family's health, so I have never felt the need to have any additional insurance.

Expert tip: When starting a new job, look carefully at the employer's health plan. You may find that TRICARE offers superior coverage at lower cost. You can decline the employer's plan and avoid payroll deductions for health care. Take the money you save and put it towards your 401k.

Public Law 109-364, Section 707 prohibits employers from enticing TRICARE-eligible employees to decline the company health plan. However, you are free to decline on your own and use TRICARE instead. Many people blindly sign up for the employer plan because they may not know they have a choice.

TRICARE Supplements

A supplement is a policy that reimburses your TRICARE deductibles and copayments. Because of its limited scope, a supplement is <u>not</u> considered to be OHI and TRICARE remains first payer. Supplements are generally quite affordable.

Just like buying comprehensive health insurance, this is a highly personal decision. Our view is that most families will not need a supplement because out-of-pocket costs with TRICARE are often quite low. What you are actually covering with a supplement are your copayments up to the limit of your catastrophic cap. Most families don't come close to reaching their cap in any given year, so a supplement just isn't worth the cost.

We can see one case where it would make sense to buy a supplement: a non-active duty family with predictably high medical expenses each year. If a family member has high recurring medical or prescription costs due to a chronic condition, then it might make sense to purchase a supplement for that individual. You can find an excellent checklist of the questions that you should ask when shopping for a supplemental policy at **www.tricare.mil/Plans/OHI/SuppInsurance**

Travel Insurance

The term "travel insurance" can mean many different things. Depending upon context, it can refer to reimbursement of travel expenses such as lost luggage, missed flights or canceled reservations. It can refer to repatriation flights/air ambulance or medical coverage for the international traveler. When discussing travel insurance, make sure everyone is talking about the same thing. In this discussion, we use the term "travel insurance" to refer to medical coverage for international travelers which may or may not include air ambulance or repatriation flights. See our discussion of Air Ambulance coverage in Chapter 4.

All TRICARE plans cover urgent and emergency care worldwide. See Chapter 5 for discussion on how to access these types of care for different beneficiary categories. Additionally, non-Prime plans like Select or TFL cover even routine care without the need for a referral. Despite this, many people are uncomfortable relying on TRICARE for international travel either due to their unfamiliarity with TRICARE's global coverage, personal doubt that it will really work, or their concern about having to pay a big bill upfront and wait for reimbursement. If you don't have ready access to cash or high credit card limits, this can be a legitimate concern. In some parts of the world, hospitals are cash-only, with payment up front. Ask about this before leaving the U.S. Know before you go!

A key reason that TRICARE users buy travel insurance is their belief that insurers will pay hospitals directly, alleviating the need to come up with large amounts of cash. Just be aware that not all insurers do this in all cases, and TRICARE itself may be able to send payment to foreign hospitals in the right circumstances. This is called "direct billing." (See Chapter 5 for strategies on this.) Another reason people buy travel insurance is a supposedly easier claims process. I have found that submitting claims for commercial insurance was no easier than doing a TRICARE claim, so that reason may or may not hold up.

Things to bear in mind if considering travel insurance:

- Travel policies are considered OHI. You MUST file claims first with the travel policy, after which you can file with TRICARE for any unpaid balance.

- There are strict time limits for how long a travel policy can remain in effect. A company I dealt with would do it only for 45 days at a time, making it unsuitable for full-time expats or global nomads. In contrast, TRICARE plans have no time limits overseas and no need for any additional premium payments.

Many commercial travel policies include transportation to the U.S. for medical treatment, recuperation, or the return of remains in case of death (called "repatriation"). This can be prohibitively expensive without insurance. TRICARE plans include limited provisions for air evacuation in cases of medical necessity and NO provision for repatriation. Air ambulance/medical evacuation is discussed in Chapter 4.

It is possible to buy an air evacuation policy without medical coverage; or medical coverage without air evacuation; or both as a package deal. Make sure that you know what services you are getting when shopping around.

Immigration and Visa Matters

Many nations around the world require travelers to provide proof of health insurance as a condition of entry. This might apply to tourists, resident/long-stay applicants, or student visas. Each nation specifies their own particular requirements of coverage; there is no broad set of rules that governs global travel. A letter from the insurance provider detailing your coverage may be required to obtain a visa.

To download proof of coverage, visit **TRICARE.mil** and click "I want to get proof of TRICARE coverage." Sadly, this letter gives little detail about actual coverage. While TRICARE plans do not have a cap on benefits, MHS resists putting this in writing so your host nation may not accept TRICARE as a qualifying policy. Because of the vague wording in the letter, host nations may find it unacceptable, forcing travelers to purchase a commercial policy to meet the visa requirements of the host nation.

For a vacationer, this might be just a mild annoyance; the cost for a few weeks of coverage is minimal. For those planning longer stays abroad, however, this becomes an expensive constraint. It might force one into a lifetime of third-party insurance that would be unnecessary if the host nation would accept TRICARE as creditable coverage.

Thailand, for example, requires travelers to buy insurance from an approved list of Thai vendors for certain types of visas. However, these policies are not sold to anyone over age 70 or so. Many retirees in Thailand are unable to obtain the required proof of coverage and they become essentially "trapped" in the country. They can freely use TRICARE in-country, but if they leave, they may not be allowed reentry as they cannot provide acceptable proof of coverage. All of this could be alleviated by a sentence or two in a letter from MHS detailing the coverage under their TRICARE plan.

I try to be apolitical in this book, but I find this level of bureaucratic indifference to be a slap in the face to our veterans who have served their nation with valor and distinction. Our view is that a team of skilled government lawyers should be clever enough to craft a letter that would be acceptable to foreign immigration authorities while still protecting the interests of the U.S. government. The problem could be quickly resolved if there were the organizational will to address it.

We are starting to see some success in this area. Expats in Thailand and the Philippines recently obtained detailed letters of TRICARE coverage from government employees who care enough to extend the effort. I will not share their contact information in this book since it is subject to change, and it is discourteous to publish individual contact information without permission. If you would like to learn how others have obtained a tailored letter of TRICARE coverage for visa or immigration purposes, please join our Facebook group *"TRICARE Around the World"* and we can discuss recent developments.

Until this problem is fixed, the best solution we can find is to provide all possible information about your TRICARE plan. Following the instructions in Chapter 6, print out a table of costs for your TRICARE plan as well as the letter mentioned above from TRICARE.mil. I successfully did this in Japan where we lived on a year-long volunteer visa. We assembled sufficient evidence about our coverage so that local authorities accepted TRICARE as our primary insurance, avoiding the expense of enrolling in the Japanese health care system.

TRICARE and Medicare

At age 65 (and sometimes earlier), most U.S. citizens and lawful residents become eligible for Medicare. Enrollment into Medicare Parts A and B places beneficiaries into TRICARE for Life (TFL). The combination of Medicare + TFL is a powerful health plan that offers worldwide coverage.

This is discussed in detail in Chapter 8, which should be read carefully <u>before</u> reaching Medicare age so you can be properly prepared.

TRICARE and Retirement Planning

I participate in a lot of <u>non-military</u> financial planning groups. There is one question that often comes up in discussions: ***What do you do if you want to retire early and have no employer-provided health coverage?*** The problem seems insurmountable to many non-military Americans under age 65 and can be the sole reason that people keep working even when they are otherwise ready to retire. On the open market with no subsidies, family coverage can easily exceed $1,500 per month.

Fortunately for readers of this book, you have a solution! **The lifetime benefits of TRICARE can free you from the shackles of working longer than you wish.** If you choose to retire from a second career before 65, you can do so without worrying about health insurance. This single advantage may put early retirement within your reach.

Earlier in this chapter, we demonstrated potential cost savings of $10,000 annually by relying solely on TRICARE instead of buying another plan. With average 8% returns (easily achievable in equity index funds), investing these funds could yield an additional $500,000 in 20 years – on top of any other

16

retirement benefits from your military and civilian career. For the sake of your financial security, you owe it to yourself and your family to learn how to do this.

If you are purchasing employer health coverage or any other policy, ask yourself why. In most cases, it is an unneeded expense. Fully embracing your TRICARE benefits can make the difference between early retirement, late retirement, a prosperous retirement, or perhaps no retirement at all.

Expert tip: If you are thinking of moving overseas and plan to claim Social Security in the future, **make sure that you sign up for a MySSA account <u>before</u> leaving the U.S.** You can use MySSA to track and apply for retirement benefits. Anti-fraud measures make it difficult or impossible to create an online account while overseas. Learn more about creating a MySSA account at **www.ssa.gov/myaccount**

Flexible Spending Accounts

Starting in 2024, changes to the U.S. tax code allow for Flexible Spending Accounts (FSA) for active duty members and certain activated Guard and Reservists. An FSA lets you set aside pre-tax money from your paycheck each month to put towards medical and dental expenses that are not otherwise covered. This reduces your taxes while giving you funds for things like copayments, deductibles, chiropractic care, dental, OTC meds, and more. Visit **www.fsafeds.gov** for details and to sign up.

Basic Cost Terms

A working knowledge of vocabulary is essential when discussing any health plan. A great deal of confusion arises when someone misuses a term like "deductible" or "copay", which can lead to costly mistakes. Please study these definitions carefully.

Premium: A recurring payment for insurance coverage that is paid monthly, quarterly, or annually. Premiums are risk-based, meaning the insurer charges enough to fully cover health expenses for their customers.

Example: TRICARE Young Adult (TYA) is a premium-based plan. By law, TYA is not subsidized with tax dollars. Premiums are adjusted annually to reflect the insurer's actual cost of providing beneficiary care, making TYA considerably more expensive than other TRICARE plans.

Fee: A recurring payment to join an insurance plan. Fee-based plans are government-subsidized, meaning that much of the cost is covered by tax dollars. Fees differ from premiums in that a fee covers only certain administrative costs of the insurer, whereas premiums cover the full cost of providing health care.

Example: TRICARE Select is fee-based. The cost is low because Select is financed (subsidized) by tax dollars.

Deductible: The amount in medical bills that one must pay before insurance benefits kick in. It is calculated on an annual basis and resets to zero at the start of each calendar year. Until the deductible is met, beneficiaries pay the full cost of care. Once the deductible is reached, insurance starts to cover the cost of care. It is calculated on a "per year" basis, not "per claim."

Example: In 2025, there is a $150 deductible for Group A retirees on Select. Benefits begin after your allowable expenses exceed $150. TRICARE Prime has zero deductible meaning that Prime benefits start with the very first dollar spent.

Copayment or copay: A fixed dollar amount that you pay for a covered service or drug.

Example: In 2025, the cost of in-network Urgent Care for a Group A retiree on Select is $37. Since this is a fixed dollar amount, it is called a copayment.

Cost-Share: A percentage of the total cost that you pay for a covered service. The percentage depends on the status of the sponsor, status of the beneficiary, the care that is obtained, and which plan is being used.

Example: The cost for the same Urgent Care mentioned above would be 25 percent of the bill, if visiting a non-network provider. As a percentage of the bill, it is called a cost-share.

Catastrophic cap: This is the most that an individual or family will pay out of pocket in a given calendar year for covered services.

Example: A Group A retiree family on Prime will have an annual catastrophic cap of $3000 in 2025. After a family pays this amount in copayments, deductibles, and fees, all remaining allowable expenses will be covered 100 percent by TRICARE for the rest of the calendar year. All TRICARE plans have a catastrophic cap except for the Point of Service (POS) option under TRICARE Prime.

Recurring fees paid for fee-based plans count towards the annual cap. Premiums for premium-based plans do not. Medicare fees also do not count.

Allowable charges: The maximum amount TRICARE will pay for a procedure or service. This amount may vary by location, TRICARE plan, and category of beneficiary (active duty vs. retiree). This is also known as CHAMPUS Maximum Allowable Charge (CMAC). Any procedure that is not covered by TRICARE, such as acupuncture, is considered "non-allowable" and would not be covered at all.

To learn more TRICARE terms and definitions, visit **https://tricare.mil/Costs/Cost-Terms**

2
Who is Covered?

WITH NEARLY 9.5 MILLION ELIGIBLE BENEFICIARIES, TRICARE is one of the nation's largest health plans. This chapter discusses the different categories of beneficiaries, what plans they are eligible for, and under what circumstances.

The first step for enrolling in TRICARE is registration in **DEERS: The Defense Enrollment Eligibility Reporting System.** DEERS is the database which lists everyone entitled to military benefits: family members, retirees, reservists, survivors, and so on. **No one can enroll in TRICARE until they are <u>first</u> registered in DEERS** (although newborns have a grace period; see below). Guidelines on how to register in DEERS can be found at **tricare.mil/requireddocuments**

If you have questions about eligibility, call your TRICARE regional contractor or the DEERS support office at 1-800-538-9552. You may also visit the DEERS/ID office at any military base. Many U.S. embassies around the world have a DEERS office who might be able to help. You will have to inquire locally to find them and learn how to visit them; however, not all DEERS locations are accessible to retirees.

Eligibility

Broadly speaking, TRICARE is a health care program for:
- Active duty military
- Military retirees including medical retirees
- Spouses and qualifying former spouses, including same sex spouses
- Surviving family members of deceased sponsors

- National Guard and Reservists (depending on category and activation status)
- Active and retired members of Coast Guard, U.S. Public Health Service, and the National Oceanic and Atmospheric Administration (NOAA)
- Minor children, adult children (to age 26), and adult children with disabilities with possible lifetime benefits
- Adopted children, stepchildren, wards, and children of unmarried parents
- Dependent parents and in-laws (limited care at participating MTFs under TRICARE Plus)
- Medal of Honor recipients and their family members
- Foreign Force Members in the U.S. on military orders.

The remainder of this chapter discusses specific eligibility criteria for each of these categories.

Uniformed Service Members

All active members of the uniformed services are covered by TRICARE. This includes U.S. Coast Guard, officers of the U.S. Public Health Service (USPHS) and of the National Oceanic and Atmospheric Administration (NOAA).

Active Duty Service Members (ADSM) are covered for medical care in nearly all situations and should never incur costs for care. They will be enrolled in TRICARE Prime or Prime Remote, depending on the proximity of the nearest MTF. There are instances where an ADSM might have to pay a bill upfront, such as in a remote location where no MTF or network provider is available, but these expenses will be fully reimbursed after they are submitted to the regional contractor.

If an ADSM receives care outside of a military hospital or clinic, they must notify their PCM at the earliest opportunity in accordance with DoD and Service regulations.

Retirees and Medically Retired

For retirees, coverage is continuous from the day you retire, but it is not automatic; **you must enroll in a plan.** The same holds true for those who are medically retired. If you hold a retiree ID card, you are eligible for TRICARE coverage, but you must enroll in a plan.

The mechanics of shifting from your active duty plan to a retiree plan can be complicated. You first must ensure that DEERS is updated to reflect the sponsor's retiree status, and this can only be done when your separating command has submitted the required paperwork. Not all personnel offices are equally efficient, so this paperwork may not be complete by your final day of active service.

Once DEERS reflects the sponsor's status as a retiree, family members can obtain retiree ID cards. After that, contact your regional contractor to enroll in a plan. Ideally, this would all happen the day after retirement, but things don't always go so smoothly. Either way, do not fear – you have 90 days from your retirement date to complete your TRICARE enrollment. Any medical expenses incurred during those 90 days will be honored. If you miss the 90-day deadline, contact your regional contractor to request a retroactive enrollment. They can backdate enrollment to your retirement date, but you will have to pay any fees that you missed. If you retire overseas, this will be even more complicated. Factor in the logistics of gaining access to a DEERS office without a valid ID card which can be an issue in some locations. Chapter 3 provides a more complete discussion of the sign-up process.

If you are in a remote overseas location with no practical way of obtaining an ID card in-country, call TRICARE Overseas as soon as DEERS reflects your retiree status. It's possible that they can enroll you in a TRICARE plan even without an ID card. Most foreign non-network healthcare providers are uninterested in your military ID, so an ID card may not be necessary for using your benefits abroad.

If you are retired from the reserves but not yet drawing retired pay (gray area retiree), you may enroll in TRICARE Retired Reserve until age 60. At age 60, transition to Prime or Select, which have much more favorable pricing.

At age 65, all retirees transition to TRICARE for Life (TFL). This requires enrollment in Medicare Parts A & B. Even if you live overseas where Medicare cannot be used, you MUST be in Medicare if you want TRICARE benefits to continue after age 65. There are some limited exceptions to this rule; please see Chapter 8 for a complete explanation.

Spouse

The spouse of a TRICARE sponsor is always eligible for TRICARE. Even if legally separated, the spouse remains eligible until divorce or annulment is finalized and perhaps even beyond that. Read the section below about former spouses, if applicable. Coverage for same-sex spouses became law on June 26, 2013, starting with the date that the spouse is registered in DEERS.

There is no requirement for spouses to be in the same TRICARE plan as their sponsor. While an active duty sponsor must be in either Prime or Prime Remote, there is no such requirement for the spouse. Run the Plan Finder Tool at **tricare.mil** to find all the plan options for spouses. You can also visit our YouTube channel **@thetricareguy.** Episode 10 has tips and tricks for getting the most from the Plan Finder Tool.

Former Spouse

The former spouse of a military sponsor may be eligible for either transitional or lifetime TRICARE coverage. There are two rules that govern eligibility of a former spouse. If neither of these rules apply, the former spouse will be eligible for transitional benefits under Continued Health Care Benefit Program (CHCBP). Benefits will be lost if the former spouse remarries or enrolls in an employer-sponsored health plan.

- **Under the 20/20/20 rule,** the former spouse can keep TRICARE benefits **indefinitely** if: (1) married to the service member for at least 20 years; (2) the service member served in the armed forces for at least 20 years; and (3) the marriage and the period of service overlapped for at least 20 years.

- **Under the 20/20/15 rule,** the former spouse may keep their TRICARE benefits for **one year after the divorce** if: (1) married to the service member for at least 20 years; (2) the service member served in the armed forces for at least 20 years; and (3) the marriage and the period of service overlapped for at least 15 years.

If the above qualifications are not met, the former spouse may apply for CHCBP, providing up to 36 months of coverage. See Chapter 7 for more about CHCBP.

A former spouse who retains TRICARE benefits will become their own sponsor in DEERS, no longer relying on their military spouse for eligibility. To establish benefits after dissolution of the marriage, they must ensure that DEERS is updated and enroll in a plan under their own sponsorship. This is done by visiting the nearest DEERS office with the marriage certificate, divorce decree, statement of military service, and two current forms of government ID. The DEERS technician will forward this information to the appropriate service component for approval. Once approved, the former spouse can get a new ID card and then enroll in a TRICARE plan. This process can be time-consuming, so start right away to make sure that you will have coverage when needed. Any eligible children from the marriage will remain under the service member sponsor for eligibility, regardless of custody arrangements.

Foreign Spouse Over 65

After age 65, virtually the only path to remain in TRICARE is to enroll in Medicare Part B, pay the monthly fee, and transition into TRICARE for Life (TFL). For most Americans, Medicare Part A is provided at no cost.

It is a bit more complicated for a foreign-born spouse who lives outside the United States, has no Social Security Number, and no U.S. work record. Such individuals may not qualify for Part A, making enrollment in TFL impossible. The foreign spouse must apply for Medicare, get disapproved, and use that notice of disapproval to continue enrollment in Select even past age 65. This is a rare loophole that many eligible spouses are unaware of. **Please see the section on "Non-U.S. Spouse" in Chapter 8** for details on how to do this.

Newborns

The newborn of a TRICARE sponsor is temporarily enrolled into TRICARE at birth. **Those born stateside** in a Prime Service Area (PSA) will be automatically enrolled into Prime. All others will be placed into Select.

The newborn's temporary TRICARE enrollment ends 90 days after birth. You must register your child in DEERS and enroll in a TRICARE plan to maintain ongoing care. You have 90 days in the U.S. or 120 days overseas to enroll your newborn in DEERS. **Any claims for care after that cutoff will be denied if your newborn is not in DEERS.** If you miss the deadline, your child will be placed into a status of Direct Care Only (DCO) until the next Open Season (enrollment window). DCO does **not** provide a full range of health care services and may, in fact, provide no services at all. You do NOT want your child to be in this status. An explanation of DCO can be found in Chapter 7.

For a child born overseas, you will need a Consular Report of Birth Abroad (CRBA, Form FS-240) to enter your child into DEERS. This document certifies that your child acquired U.S. citizenship at birth. The American Citizen Services (ACS) unit of the nearest embassy will be able to help. The child does not need a Social Security Number (SSN) to register, but their DEERS information should be updated once they have one.

Tips for enrolling newborns into TRICARE can be found at **www.tricare.mil/LifeEvents/Baby/GettingTRICAREforChild**

Minor Children

Unmarried biological children, stepchildren, and adopted children of sponsors are eligible for TRICARE until age 21 (or age 23 if enrolled full-time in an accredited institution of higher learning). Beyond that, eligible unmarried adult children can enroll in TRICARE Young Adult until age 26. (See the following section on Adult Children.)

Other provisions for children include:

- **Unadopted stepchildren** are eligible for TRICARE benefits only if the parent of the child is married to the sponsor. If the marriage terminates, stepchildren lose eligibility on the date of the final decree.

- If the sponsor **adopts his or her stepchildren**, they remain covered even if the marriage ends.

- **Adult children of TRICARE sponsors who have a serious disability that began prior to age 21** remain eligible for the duration of the disability. See the section below on Adult Children with Disabilities.

- **Children whose sponsor died while serving on active duty** remain eligible for TRICARE until they lose eligibility due to age, marriage, or other reason. See the section below about survivors of deceased sponsors.

The Ultimate Guide to TRICARE

In other scenarios, children also may be eligible for TRICARE:

- If born out of wedlock.
- When placed in the custody of a sponsor, either by a court or recognized agency, as a ward, or in anticipation of adoption.

In each case, there are amplifying rules and conditions. Contact your regional contractor to learn if your child qualifies. The prerequisite for any beneficiary is to enroll them in DEERS. If you are near a military base, the DEERS/ID office will be able to help. In some countries, you might be able to find a DEERS office associated with the U.S. embassy or at the Joint U.S. Military Advisory Group (JUSMAG), normally affiliated with the embassy.

Adult Children

Adult children age out of your TRICARE plan at age 21, or at 23 if they are enrolled full time in college. If you are claiming the extension to age 23, you will need a letter from the school's registrar confirming your child's enrollment. Annual renewal of this letter may be required by your regional contractor. Following the age cutoff, unmarried adult children under age 26 are eligible for TRICARE Young Adult (TYA) if the child does not have access to their own employer-sponsored health plan. TYA has two variants: **TYA-Prime** and **TYA-Select**. Your adult child may also participate in the U.S. Family Health Plan (USFHP) if they live in a region where this is offered. These plans are described in Chapter 7.

TYA is a premium-based plan. This means it is not subsidized with tax dollars, making the cost more comparable to commercial health plans. It might pay to compare with plans in your state health insurance marketplace. You can get more details by visiting **tricare.mil/Plans/HealthPlans/TYA**

Adult Children with Disabilities

Incapacitated or significantly disabled adult children of sponsors may be eligible to remain in TRICARE throughout their lifetime if they meet the following criteria:

- Incapable of providing their own support
- Dependent on the sponsor for over 50 percent of their support. If the sponsor is deceased, the child must have been receiving over 50 percent of his or her support from the sponsor at the time of death.
- Incapacitation must have occurred prior to age 21 (or age 23 if enrolled as a full-time student).
- The adult child must be unmarried. If they marry and the marriage ends due to divorce, annulment, or death of the spouse, TRICARE benefits may be reinstated if all other requirements are still met.

The application and approval process can be prolonged, so start well before the 21st birthday to avoid a break in coverage. If you miss this deadline, benefits may be applied retroactively as long as you can demonstrate that the disability occurred before the 21st birthday. The following documentation is required:

- Dependency Statement — Incapacitated Child Over Age 21 (DD Form 137-5)
- Application for Identification Card/DEERS Enrollment (DD Form 1172-2)
- Current physician's statement dated within 90 days. Contact the sponsor's service representative for details.
- If the child is eligible for Medicare Part A, include proof of Medicare Part A and Part B enrollment unless the sponsor is on active duty. If not eligible for Part A, submit a statement from SSA certifying non-eligibility.
- Birth certificate, if not enrolled in DEERS. If adding a stepchild to DEERS, the parents' marriage certificate is also required.

Recertification of the disability is required every four years to maintain benefits. This is something that should be planned for if the adult child has custodial arrangements following the death of their parents. They can maintain TRICARE throughout their lifetime provided this four-year recertification continues without interruption.

In Chapter 14, we provide tips and information on lifetime care for adult children with severe disabilities. Additional resources are listed at **www.militaryonesource.mil/family-relationships/special-needs**

Guard and Reserve Members

TRICARE eligibility for National Guard, Reservists, and their family members varies depending on several factors. **Always use the Plan Finder Tool separately** for the sponsor and for each family member to determine which plans apply to each person. Go to **tricare.mil/Plans/PlanFinder**

A National Guard or Reserve member who has been activated for more than 30 days on **Federal orders** (Title 10) may be eligible for the same TRICARE plans as active duty members, including their dependents. For Guard members activated on **State orders** (Title 32), there is no TRICARE eligibility.

Reservists who are in a full-time position, drawing full military pay and benefits, will be enrolled in TRICARE Prime or Prime Remote, depending on proximity to the nearest MTF. Their eligible family members can also enroll in these plans, as well as Select and U.S. Family Health Plan, if available.

Under age 60, retired Reserve members may purchase **TRICARE Retired Reserve,** a premium-based plan. This includes family members and survivors of deceased sponsors if the sponsor was covered by TRICARE Retired Reserve when he or she died. See Chapter 7 for more information or visit **tricare.mil/Plans/HealthPlans/TRR**

Members of the **Selected Reserve** may be eligible for **TRICARE Reserve Select (TRS)** if they are not on active duty orders and are not covered by the Transitional Assistance Management Program (TAMP) or Federal Employees Health Benefits (FEHB). For more details on TRS, read Chapter 7 or visit **tricare.mil/Plans/HealthPlans/TRS**

When the retired reservist turns 60, they and their dependents become eligible for the same TRICARE plans as regular retired service members. This includes TRICARE Prime, TRICARE Select, and U.S. Family Health Plan (USFHP).

At age 65, retired Reservists become eligible for **TRICARE for Life**. They will need to enroll in and pay for Medicare Part B to continue their TRICARE coverage. Their dependent family members under age 65 will continue on their other plans until they, too, reach age 65. Chapter 8 has a full discussion of TRICARE for Life and Medicare.

Members of the **Individual Ready Reserve** (IRR) are not eligible for any TRICARE coverage.

Survivors of Deceased Sponsors

Surviving family members of deceased sponsors can retain their TRICARE benefits depending upon the sponsor's military status when they passed. Spouses lose eligibility when they remarry and do not regain coverage if that subsequent marriage terminates. See **tricare.mil/Plans/Eligibility/Survivors** for full details.

Visit **tricare.mil** and use the **Plan Finder Tool** to determine suitable plans for a surviving spouse and children. For the first question, **select "Surviving Spouse" or "Surviving Child"** rather than "Spouse" or "Child." When it later asks for sponsor status, select their status at the time of death. Answer all the remaining questions to see which plans each family member is eligible for.

The spouse of a sponsor who dies while on active duty is considered a "transitional survivor" for three years from the date of death.

- For the first three years following the death of their sponsor, they will have the same TRICARE benefits and pricing of an Active Duty Family Member (ADFM).

- Following that three-year period, the surviving spouse will have access to plans and pricing of a retiree family member.

Surviving children of a deceased active duty sponsor are considered to be "transitional survivors" for a three-year period, but in a different sense than the surviving spouse.

- Surviving children will have access to TRICARE plans and pricing of ADFM until they age out of TRICARE at 21 or 23.

- During that three-year transitional period, they will also have access to active duty-only programs such as the Extended Care Health Option (ECHO). After the three-year transitional period, they will lose access to these AD-only programs. The various special programs are discussed in Chapter 7.

If a sponsor dies after retiring from active duty (either regular or a medical retirement), surviving family members remain eligible for TRICARE with the same plan options and costs as before. The surviving spouse will remain eligible for TRICARE unless they remarry. Children remain eligible until they age out or lose TRICARE eligibility for other reasons, such as marriage.

Surviving family members may retain **transitional dental coverage under the TRICARE Dental Program (TDP) Survivor Benefit Plan.** A surviving spouse can remain on TDP for three years, then transition to FEDVIP dental. Children can remain on TDP until they lose eligibility at age 21 or 23. While on

TDP, survivor premiums are covered at no cost, and the beneficiary pays only their cost-share. Learn more at: **www.tricare.mil/CoveredServices/Dental/ RetireeSurvivorBenefit**

Medal of Honor Recipients & Their Families

Medal of Honor (MoH) recipients and their TRICARE-eligible family members have somewhat expanded access to TRICARE as compared to other members.

- If a non-retired MoH recipient **separates** from the service, then the sponsor and their family members retain the TRICARE benefits of a **retired** sponsor.

- If the sponsor is **retired or on active duty**, then they and their family members will have the same TRICARE benefits as other retired or active duty sponsors.

- If the MoH recipient is **deceased**, surviving eligible family members will retain the TRICARE benefits of survivors of deceased active duty or retired sponsors, depending on whether the sponsor was on active duty or not at the time of death.

See the previous section on "Survivors of Deceased Sponsors" for further explanation of survivor benefits.

Dependent Parents

If you have dependent parents or in-laws, they may be eligible for limited TRICARE benefits. "Dependent" means that the sponsor is providing more than half of the parent's living expenses. The parent must be enrolled in DEERS, and evidence of financial support will be required when applying.

The only plan that a dependent parent can enroll in is TRICARE Plus. This plan has strict limitations. It can be used only at participating MTFs and provides priority access for Primary Care <u>only</u>. Specialty care within an MTF is not assured, and **no coverage is provided off base**. Acceptance into TRICARE Plus at one MTF is not transferable to another location. If the dependent parent is not near an MTF, this coverage is basically unusable. It is important to understand that even in the best case, TRICARE Plus is for primary care only; it does not assure access to specialty care. It should not be viewed as a full-service health plan; the dependent parent will still need another form of full-service health care. See Chapter 7 for more information about TRICARE Plus.

3
Selecting & Enrolling in a Plan

DECIDING WHICH PLAN TO ENROLL IN can seem daunting. There are so many unfamiliar concepts: Managed vs. self-directed care. Premiums, deductibles, and copayments. In-network, non-network, PCMs, and referrals. Hopefully, the previous chapters have provided clarity to some of these terms.

In this chapter, we walk through the decision-making process so that you can choose the plan that best meets your needs. We also explain how and when you can sign up. We have several YouTube videos on this subject and, as always, our Facebook groups are available to interact with the author and a supportive community of TRICARE users. To find our online resources, visit **www.theTRICAREguy.com**

Step 1: Use the Plan Finder Tool

When deciding on which plan to choose for you and your family, the best place to start is the TRICARE Plan Finder tool. This can be found on the official TRICARE website by clicking "Plans" at the top of the page.

If the sponsor is active duty, make sure to run this tool <u>twice</u>: once for the sponsor and again for eligible family members. Also run it for each family member if you are geographically separated because you may get differing results based on location. Family members do not all have to be in the same plan. If you are planning ahead for military retirement, run the tool as though you are already retired to see which plans it will recommend for you as a former/retired military member. Put in your retirement ZIP Code, if known, and retiree status for more relevant results. This can help you anticipate your plan choices in retirement. Visit our YouTube channel for a video on using the Plan Finder Tool to conduct "what-if" scenarios.

The simplest outcome is when the Plan Finder identifies only one available plan. In that case, you have no choice but to enroll in that plan. It is quite possible that the tool will identify two or more possible plans, in which case you will have to dig a bit deeper to see which plan best fits your needs. Cost and details of each plan are discussed in Chapters 6 & 7.

Here are some possible outcomes from the Plan Finder tool and how you might respond:

- Active Duty members will always be directed to TRICARE Prime or Prime Remote, depending on their proximity to an MTF. These are managed-care plans for which you will be assigned a Primary Care Manager (PCM).

- Active Duty Family Members (ADFM) do NOT have to be in the same plan as their sponsor. Many in our Facebook group have said that they were falsely told by TRICARE Overseas that they MUST enroll in Prime, even though they preferred to be in Select. **Do not let them force you into a plan that you don't want!** Family members can be in Select if that is their preference. If Prime or Prime Remote is available in your area, the Plan Finder tool will let you know.

- There may also be an option for the **U.S. Family Health Plan** if it is available near you. USFHP is a form of TRICARE Prime, offered by certain regional health care networks within the United States. Carefully review the USFHP plan near you to help in your decision-making process. Plans are listed at **USFHP.com**

- If you do not live in a Prime Service Area (PSA), you will not be offered TRICARE Prime. There is a provision for signing a waiver to accept Prime despite living a long distance from an MTF. We have consistently found dissatisfaction among our group members who do this. Think about it: You are accepting a plan that is <u>not</u> offered in your area AND you will have great difficulty in finding providers and getting referrals within a reasonable driving distance. If you do not live in a PSA and are not an active duty member, you should strongly lean towards TRICARE Select. After a short learning curve, you will likely be quite happy with this choice.

- Retirees and their family members cannot enroll in TRICARE Prime Overseas. Do not try to "spoof" the system by enrolling in Stateside Prime while living overseas; the process of obtaining referrals will be unmanageable, making your health benefits extremely hard to use.

- Any beneficiary over age 65 will be directed to TRICARE for Life (TFL). Enrollment in Medicare Part B is required, including the monthly Medicare fee that goes with it. If you are <u>under</u> 65 and eligible for Medicare due to a qualifying medical condition, you may be given a choice of TFL, Prime or Select. Those under 65 may lose access to Medicare once the qualifying medical condition is alleviated. See Chapter 8 for information about TFL and Medicare.

There is an option called **TRICARE Plus**. Plus is an add-on to non-managed plans such as TRICARE Select or TFL. The Plan Finder Tool will never recommend Plus except for dependent parents and in-laws, for whom this is the only available plan. TRICARE Plus offers primary care at participating MTFs, but it does <u>not</u> ensure access to specialty care and will not cover <u>any</u> care from civilian providers. **No one should rely on Plus as their sole health plan because it does not provide comprehensive care.** Learn more about this in Chapter 7.

Step 2: Evaluate Your Options

Once you run the Plan Finder Tool, it's time to decide which plan best meets your needs. Should you choose TRICARE Prime, which has higher monthly fees but no deductible? Should you choose TRICARE Select, which has a lower monthly fee but higher copayments and no PCM?

TRICARE provides two additional tools to help with this decision. These tools allow you to examine plans side-by-side for an easier comparison of costs and benefits:

- The Plan Comparison Tool, which is found at **tricare.mil/Plans/ComparePlans**
- The Cost Tool at **tricare.mil/CompareCosts**

When comparing two plans, consider your family's typical usage of health care. Which cost structure appeals to you more and is likely to save you the most money? An even bigger consideration may be this: **Under TRICARE Prime, you are assigned a Primary Care Manager (PCM)** who will be your first stop for most care. Only with their referral can you be seen by a specialist. Many people find comfort in being under the care of a PCM who guides their health care choices.

Under TRICARE Select, you do NOT have a PCM. You make appointments as you see fit and do not need referrals to see a specialist. Many people prefer the freedom of making their own health care choices without the added step of visiting a PCM and waiting for approval of their referrals.

Many new retiree families shy away from Select due to its unfamiliarity or perception that it is a "lesser" plan. The author has been enrolled in TRICARE Select as a retiree in Japan, Thailand, and Hawaii, and it has worked well in all settings. We could just pick the specialist we needed and go. There were no network providers in our overseas locations, so we paid up-front and became proficient in the art of filing claims (see Chapters 12

and 13). In Hawaii, we found plenty of network providers and
have never had to file a claim there. All in all, we've been very
pleased with TRICARE Select. Join our Facebook group to
discuss this further.

Know your rights! Military spouses in Germany, Guam,
and Australia have stated that they were "forced" into Prime
against their wishes. They were told by TRICARE Overseas that
they had to choose Prime, even though they preferred Select. We
believe these members were misinformed. The only ones who
<u>must</u> use Prime (or Prime Remote) are active duty military
members. All others who are eligible for Prime may enroll in
Select, if they so choose. If you find yourself being forced into a
plan that you don't want, push back! There are no right or wrong
answers to your choice of plans. It is a personal decision, not
always a matter of dollars and cents. Sometimes, being able to
see the doctor of your choice may be more important than
deductibles and copayments.

Real Life Story: Prime vs. Select

A member of our Facebook group shared this story of
medical treatment under Prime vs. Select. We do not claim that
this is representative of all cases, but it offers food for thought
when comparing plans. Her post is edited for brevity:

> Several years ago, my daughter (on Select) and a friend's
> daughter (on Prime) both injured their backs in gymnastics.
>
> On Select, my daughter skipped her PCP and went straight to
> a sports medicine orthopedist. She had an x-ray in the office,
> then an MRI the same day at an imaging center. The next day,
> she started Physical Therapy (PT) three times per week.
>
> On Prime, my friend's daughter had to visit her PCM. He
> ordered x-rays, which were done the same day. Two days
> later, he received the report and decided that she needed to
> go to a specialist and put in a referral. Five days later the

referral was approved, and an appointment was scheduled for about a week later. At that appointment, an MRI was ordered, which also had to be authorized. Several days later, the MRI was approved and scheduled for three weeks later. They asked for a quicker appointment, which was denied since her condition didn't require immediate medical attention. MRI received, and back to the specialist, who ordered PT. It was decided that he couldn't order PT; it had to go back to the PCM. After that appointment, PT was ordered and started.

Six weeks had passed. My daughter was nearly recovered after six weeks of PT, and her friend was just starting.

Step 3: Take Care of All Family Members

When selecting a TRICARE plan, it is important to consider all family members. Each must be individually enrolled; it is not automatic. Some key points to keep in mind:

- **Family members do not have to be in the same plan.** There are many situations in which different members would benefit from being in different plans. Talk this over with your regional contractor.
- **Creating an account in your regional web portal is NOT the same as enrolling in a plan**. To enroll your family in a TRICARE plan, call your regional contractor. It can all be done over the phone, including setting up monthly payments.
- **There are only specific times of the year when you may enroll in a plan:** Either during the annual Open Season or when you have a Qualifying Life Event (QLE). If you miss these opportunities, you may have to wait an entire year before you get another chance. See the next section for information about this.

Due to medical privacy laws, TRICARE will not talk to you about your spouse or adult children without pre-authorization. Use DD Form 2870 (Authorization for Disclosure of Medical or

Dental Information) to provide this authorization. Or, with TRICARE Overseas, create online accounts for each family member and link the accounts in the web portal. **This linking of accounts grants permission** for you to discuss your family member's medical care and enrollment. Appendix A includes instructions for linking accounts and managing family health plans in the regional contractor web portals.

Expert tip: Linkage to a child's account expires on their 18th birthday. If you want to remain involved in the management of your adult child's health care, they must reestablish consent after they turn 18.

Open Season and QLEs: When to Sign Up

There are two main opportunities to make changes to your family's TRICARE enrollment: during the annual Open Season and after a Qualifying Life Event (QLE). If you miss those time frames, other ways to change enrollment are described below.

Open Season, sometimes called the **Annual Enrollment Window**, takes place each year from mid-November to mid-December. Check **tricare.mil** or our Facebook group for exact dates. During Open Season, all TRICARE beneficiaries can make changes to their enrollment, if desired. This can be done with a phone call to your regional contractor or via their web portal. **Any changes made during Open Season will be effective on January 1st of the following year.** Phone lines can be quite busy during this period, so call as early as possible in the enrollment period.

If you do not need to make changes to your plan, you normally do not have to call or take any action during Open Season. However, this is not always true: An exception came in the fall of 2020 when a new fee was initiated for many retirees enrolled in TRICARE Select. To retain coverage, affected members had to arrange payment for the new fee during the

2020 Open Season even though they were not changing plans. So, while the general rule is that you do not need to call if you are not changing plans, watch out for exceptions to the rule.

The other opportunity to switch TRICARE plans is when **anyone** in your family has a **Qualifying Life Event (QLE)**. Any change made as the result of a QLE becomes effective as of the date of the event. For example, if you got married on April 1st and notified TRICARE on April 20th, any medical expenses incurred by your new spouse would be covered back to April 1st. You generally have **90 days** from the QLE to notify TRICARE of the change. Failure to do so might mean that you will have to wait for the next Open Season to make the enrollment change.

A complete list of QLEs with examples is shown below. You can learn more about TRICARE Qualifying Life Events at **tricare.mil/LifeEvents**

- **Change in sponsor status.** Examples: Retiring or separating from active duty; Reserve activation or deactivation.

- **Change in family composition.** Examples: Marriage, divorce, or annulment; birth or adoption of a child; guardianship; death in the family.

- **Moving.** Examples: Relocation to a new TRICARE region; an eligible child moving away to college.

- **Government-directed changes.** Example: A government-directed change of your primary care manager or plan.

- **Change in overseas command sponsorship.** Example: Gaining or losing permission to have family members accompany sponsor during an overseas assignment.

- **Age-related changes.** Examples: Retired Reserve member turning 60; reaching Medicare age at 65; adult child losing eligibility at 21 or 23.

- **Gaining or losing Other Health Insurance (OHI).**
  Examples: Gaining or losing employer-sponsored health insurance.

If <u>any</u> member of your family has a QLE, then <u>every</u> member of the family has 90 days to change plans. For example, if the sponsor reaches age 65 and signs up for Medicare/TFL, then <u>all</u> family members are in a QLE and have 90 days to change plans, if desired.

There are two additional opportunities to change your family's TRICARE plans:

- If you want to enroll in a premium-based plan, you may do so at any time. A premium-based plan is one that is not subsidized with tax dollars and members bear the full cost of health care through premiums. This includes TRICARE Young Adult, TRICARE Reserve Select, and TRICARE Retired Reserve.

- You can request to change plans when you have a unique family situation by asking your regional contractor for an **Exception to Policy (ETP)**. A military spouse living in Germany, for example, might want to switch from TRICARE Prime to Select to have a greater choice of prenatal care off base. **Approval of ETP is not assured. If this is important to you, submit your request early and provide justification.**

TRICARE Overseas vs. Stateside Plans

In our Facebook groups, some retired members have mentioned living overseas full time while remaining in TRICARE Prime with TRICARE East or West rather than enrolling in TRICARE Overseas Select. They believe that they are deriving greater benefit through this strategy, but we disagree for the reasons below. (This does <u>not</u> apply to vacationers, who should remain enrolled in their stateside plan while traveling abroad.)

- If you are enrolled in TRICARE Overseas Select or TRICARE for Life, you can obtain all care – even for routine matters – without pre-approval. These plans have no Primary Care Manager (PCM), so obtaining care overseas is vastly simpler.

- TRICARE Prime has higher monthly fees than TRICARE Overseas Select. These fees add up, especially if you do not use your benefits very often.

- If you are enrolled in TRICARE Prime stateside and seek routine care overseas, you must have pre-approval or a referral from your PCM in the U.S. The logistics for making this request are complicated, and there is no guarantee that your request will be approved.

- It can be difficult or impossible to find an in-network provider overseas, which means your costs under Prime may be higher than you expect.

- If you obtain routine care with Prime without a referral, you will be charged the Point of Service (POS) rate, which is very costly. Your copay is 50 percent in addition to a special deductible of $300 per person. None of the costs under the POS option count towards your annual Catastrophic Cap, so there is no limit to your out-of-pocket costs. Learn more about the Point of Service option in Chapter 7, under TRICARE Prime.

- If you are in TRICARE Prime and seek emergency care overseas – which should normally be covered – there is always a chance that the claims adjudicator will decide that your condition was not a true emergency. If this happens, you could be liable for the 50 percent POS copayment and/or a long battle to dispute the claim. If you are enrolled in TRICARE Select, this would not happen because you can seek all types of care under Select without pre-approval, whether it is urgent, emergency, or routine care.

Remaining enrolled in a stateside Prime plan while living overseas potentially introduces problems and risks. It is much better – in the author's opinion – for retiree members living overseas to enroll in an overseas plan.

4
Covered Care

TRICARE HEALTH PLANS OFFER A BROAD RANGE OF SERVICES for beneficiaries. The TRICARE website says: *"TRICARE covers services that are medically necessary and considered proven."* It goes on to explain that *"medically necessary means it is appropriate, reasonable, and adequate for your condition."*

In general, the criteria for obtaining care with TRICARE is:

- Is the care medically necessary?
- Is the treatment appropriate for the disease or condition?
- Is it a proven treatment?

If the answer is yes to all three questions, there's a good chance the procedure is covered. When in doubt it is best to confirm this ahead of time. We will explain how this process work.

Covered Care Search Tool

The TRICARE website does not have any specific list of what is covered. Instead, you use the Covered Care Search Tool. Visit **tricare.mil** and click on "What's Covered" at the top. Type a word or phrase in the search box and click "Search." This will bring up a list of related topics with a discussion of how or whether they are covered by TRICARE. You also have the option to browse by category such as Primary Care, Specialty Care, etc.

In the search results, the tool displays a table showing types of care related to your search. You have to be careful at this point, or you might reach the wrong conclusion. The second column of the table – labeled "Covered?" – will say either "Yes", "No", or "It Depends." *This is highly misleading!* When the table says "Yes" or "No", don't stop at that point because it may not be the complete story! The fourth column of the table has the word "More" which is clickable. Click on "More" and you will see an amplifying page that describes when – or if – this particular type of care is covered in your situation.

Here's an example. If you search for Lung Cancer Screening, the resulting table will say "Yes": Lung cancer screening is covered. However, when you click "More", you learn that screening is limited by the age of the patient, extent of tobacco usage, and other criteria. In reality, lung cancer screening should be labeled "It depends." This disparity comes up frequently in the "What's Covered" page. Do not take "yes" or "no" at face value.

If you are unsure whether a procedure is covered, call your TRICARE regional contractor or the MHS Nurse Advice Line. If you are facing an expensive procedure and don't want any misunderstanding about your coverage, **ask your regional contractor for a "Benefits Review."** This is a formalized determination that a procedure you want is covered. **Request the review to be sent to you in writing via secure messaging to document what you were told.**

Real Life Story: Benefits Review in Germany

A member in our Facebook group was facing a cost of $89,000 for surgery at a German hospital. She called the TRICARE Overseas regional office in the UK for a benefits review, which determined that the procedure was covered. She confidently went forward with the surgery, knowing that the claim would be honored.

Before being admitted for treatment, another member in Germany was asked by their hospital for proof that TRICARE would pay for her care. TRICARE Overseas conducted a benefits review and prepared a letter listing medical codes for the covered procedures as well as details of her coverage. The hospital accepted this letter as proof of coverage and went forward with the procedure without any further issues. They used the provided medical codes, and the claim was processed with no difficulty. The benefits review process is not just for your peace of mind but can also assure the hospital that your medical expenses will be paid, so they are comfortable sending the bill to TRICARE rather than having you pay the entire bill up front.

What is NOT Covered

After settling the question of what *is* covered, you will find that determining what is *not* covered is more straightforward. There is an actual list of exclusions, which can be found at **tricare.mil/CoveredServices/IsItCovered/Exclusions.** We have chosen not to publish the list here because exclusions are subject to change. Please visit the web page above to check.

Each item on the Exclusions page is a clickable link. Click any item to learn about limitations, exceptions, or amplifying information. It is important to understand the meaning of each one. For example, skilled nursing is a covered benefit, but long term care, nursing homes, and retirement homes are not. You need to understand the difference. Clicking their links will help you understand the meaning of these different terms.

Preventive Care

TRICARE plans offer a broad range of preventive care benefits. Many preventive services are provided at no cost, meaning there is no copay and no deductible. One question we see a lot in our online forum – especially from retirees living overseas – is whether annual physicals are covered. As always, the short answer is: "It depends." But first, we must get our terminology straight.

There are physicals, wellness exams, preventive exams, and a term called Health Promotion and Disease Prevention (HP&DP) exams. Each of these is covered under different situations.

- **Physicals** are covered for active duty members, for active duty family members if required for overseas duty assignment, and for children when required for school enrollment. TRICARE does NOT cover sports physicals.

- TRICARE covers annual **Well Woman exams** at no cost. This includes breast exam, pelvic exam, Pap smear, HPV DNA testing, and other screenings when ordered or recommended during the exam.

- All TRICARE plans cover annual **Well-Child Care** at no cost until the child's 6th birthday. Services provided are listed later in this chapter.

- What used to be called a **Preventive Care Exam** is now a **Health Promotion and Disease Prevention (HP&DP) Exam**. The TRICARE cost tables say there is a copayment for this when using a non-network provider, but those living overseas often get full reimbursement for these exams in recent years, even with non-network providers. Make clear in your claim that the exam is strictly for preventive care, not for any clinical treatment.

Expert tip: If submitting a claim for an HP & DP exam, be careful how you phrase it in on the claim form. Do not write "physical" because this is not covered for most beneficiaries. Also, do not list any physical ailment in the claim, such as "monitor hypertension." If you list a physical ailment, the visit is considered clinical, not preventive, and you will have a copayment. Be sure to write only "Annual Preventive Care Exam" or "Health Promotion and Disease Prevention Exam."

During the course of the exam, it is fine to talk to your doctor about any medical issues you may have – that is the whole reason for the exam, and it will not result in denial of your claim. The doctor should schedule a follow-up appointment to deal with those medical issues at another time.

The following is a list of preventive care services covered by TRICARE. Some have exclusions or limitations. For details and a current list, visit **tricare.mil/HealthWellness/Preventive**

Abdominal Aortic Aneurysm Screening
Blood Pressure Screening
Body Measurement
Breast Exams
Breast Magnetic Resonance Imaging (MRI)
Cancer Screening
Cardiovascular Screening
Cholesterol Testing
Colonoscopy
Echocardiogram
Health Promotion & Disease Prevention Exams
Hearing Exams
Hepatitis B/C Screening
Human Papillomavirus (HPV) Test & Vaccine
Immunizations (CDC-recommended)
Infectious Disease Screening
Lipid Panel
Mammograms
Parent & Patient Educational Counseling
Pediatric Lead Level Screening
Physicals (in limited circumstances)
Rubella Antibodies
Tobacco Cessation Services
Tuberculosis Screening
Well Child Care
Well Woman Exams

Well Child Care (from birth through age 5)

Newborn care
History and physical examination
Mental health assessment
Developmental and behavioral appraisal:

Height and weight measurement
Eye & vision screening at birth and at 6 months old
Audiology screening before 1 month old
Dental Screenings
Routine immunizations
Tuberculin test at 12 months again in 2nd year of age
Hemoglobin/hematocrit testing in each of first two years
Urinalysis in each of first two years
Annual blood pressure screening age 3-6
Blood Lead Testing
Health guidance & counseling; breast feeding coaching
Routine eye exams at ages 3 and 5

Full details of well-child care can be found at **tricare.mil/CoveredServices/IsItCovered/WellChildCare**. Information on all preventive care services are listed at **tricare.mil/HealthWellness/Preventive/GettingCare**

Pharmacy

TRICARE provides comprehensive prescription drug coverage. There are various ways to receive prescriptions.

- **At an MTF at no cost**.

- **Home delivery via Express Scripts**. Express Scripts will mail only to U.S. addresses including APO or FPO overseas. **Not available in Germany,** whether by APO or German mailing address, due to German law.

- **At retail pharmacies.** This is nominally priced for a 30-day supply, but generally non-narcotic maintenance medications are provided in 90-day refills.

- **Through Accredo,** for those with complex/chronic health conditions requiring specialty medications.

- **Through the VA.** Even without any service-connected disability, many veterans can obtain prescription refills from the VA by mail or in person. See "VA Health Care" in Chapter 10.

TRICARE doesn't cover over the counter (OTC) drugs and supplies, except the following. This list is as of April 2025; use the What's Covered tool at TRICARE.mil and search for OTC to view the current list. Prescription may be required. Your local MTF might offer a wider variety of OTC medications, if it is in their formulary. For instance, we have gotten fluoride pills at no cost on base when prescribed by our child's dentist.

- Cetirizine tablets
- Fexofenadine tablets
- Certain tobacco cessation products
- Loratadine tablets
- Doxylamine 25 mg
- Levonorgestrel (Plan B Emergency Contraceptive)
- Omeprazole (generic of Prilosec OTC)

OTC medications are not covered in international locations under any circumstances.

TRICARE's pharmacy program is managed by Express Scripts. Each family member can create an account on **militaryrx.express-scripts.com** to manage prescriptions online. In the portal, members can search for participating pharmacies, order refills, check prices, set up automatic refills by mail, and see which formularies are covered under your plan.

If someone in your family has a complex or chronic health condition such as cancer, hepatitis C, HIV, or multiple sclerosis, **Accredo** may be able to provide the medications they need. Visit **www.accredo.com/dodspecialty** and read their FAQs on how to get started. At present, you can browse the list of medications on your ExpressScripts account; any that are available for delivery via Accredo will have a link to establish delivery. Call Accredo at 1-800-803-2523 for more information.

Another pharmacy benefit is the **Deployment Prescription Program (DPP)**. This allows deploying service members or TRICARE-eligible contractors and government employees (such as a military spouse or retiree) to receive up to 180 days of prescription medications while on deployment on orders. **Exception**: DPP is <u>not</u> available if you have other health insurance (OHI) with a pharmacy benefit. By law, you must use your other insurance first.

DPP also provides mail delivery to a deployment military address. Allow 3-4 weeks for the first delivery. To sign up, visit **www.militaryrx.express-scripts.com** and select DPP on the "Benefits" menu at the top.

Chapter 11 presents a number of strategies for obtaining prescription refills while traveling.

Hearing Aids

Advances in technology and changes in government regulation have led to rapid expansion in the U.S. hearing aid market in recent years. The result has been greater choice for consumers, at lower cost.

In November 2022, the U.S. Food and Drug Administration (FDA) authorized the sale of hearing aids without an audiologist. This brought a broad range of retailers and innovators into the market, slashing the cost of hearing aids by as much as 90 percent. The FDA advises that purchasing hearing aids without the involvement of an audiologist is intended only for those over 18 with mild-to-moderate hearing loss. For all others, consulting an audiologist is strongly urged as underlying issues should be investigated. Visit the FDA website for more information.

For the military community, there are a number of ways to obtain hearing aids, either through TRICARE or other means. Each of these options is explained below.

1. **Active duty service members and their families:** TRICARE can provide hearing aids if the following hearing loss thresholds are met:

- **Adults:** At least 40 dB loss in one or both ears at 500, 1000, 1500, 2000, 3000, or 4000Hz; or at least 26 dB loss in one or both ears at three or more of those frequencies; or speech recognition score less than 94%.

- **Children:** At least 26dB loss in one or both ears at 500, 1000, 2000, 3000, or 4000Hz.

Visit **tricare.mil/CoveredServices** and type "hearing aids" in the search box to learn more. If you are on TRICARE Prime, be sure to get a referral from your PCM so that your expenses will be covered.

2. **Children of Retirees:** Dependent children of retirees may be eligible for hearing aids under TRICARE. This expansion of benefits was announced in November 2024, with the following provisions:

- The child must be enrolled in Prime or USFHP
- Specific hearing loss thresholds have been met
- The recipient resides in the United States, and
- Their sponsor must still be living.

3. **The Retiree At-Cost Hearing Aid Program (RACHAP) or Retiree Hearing Aid Purchase Program (RHAPP).** Retirees (but not their family members) may be able to purchase hearing aids at greatly reduced cost at participating MTFs.

- Contact the audiology department of any MTF to see if they participate.
- Be sure to factor in the cost of travel if the MTF is not nearby; this can affect the financial benefit of this option.

4. **VA Health Care.** This option may provide hearing aids to veterans even with **no service-connected hearing loss.** Chapter 10 describes the VA Health Care Program. Read the author's real world story in the next section about obtaining hearing aids through VA Health Care.

5. Finally, you can **pay out-of-pocket** for a hearing aid purchase, either with or without the involvement of an audiologist. Many Costco locations have an onsite audiologist, offering their brand of hearing aids at a reasonable cost. Other retail outlets have similar services. Even online purchases are possible. None of this constitutes a recommendation or endorsement; we just want you to be aware of your options.

Real Life Story: Hearing Aids with VA Health Care

Chapter 10 describes the VA Health Care Program, through which veterans can obtain care even without a service-connected disability. This is my personal story of obtaining hearing aids at the VA at no cost <u>without</u> a disability rating.

When first approved for VA Health Care, I was assigned to a VA primary care physician and scheduled my first appointment. We met via video chat as many appointments were virtual during the COVID pandemic. We spent 45 minutes discussing my medical history, and she entered all my TRICARE prescriptions into the VA system for future refills by mail. No in-person exam or tests were needed.

She asked what other specialized care I would like, so I mentioned mental health counseling and help with my hearing loss. She quickly set up appointments for both. The counseling was done via video chat over multiple sessions and was extremely helpful. The hearing test was conducted two months later at the VA Medical Center in Honolulu. The audiologist confirmed my need for hearing aids and recommended a product by Oticon. I had a $50 copayment for the audiology appointment due to my VA priority group, but the hearing aids were free. From the time that I joined VA Health Care until I received my hearing aids was seven months. It would have been faster, but COVID and holidays added some delay.

All in all, it was a very good experience, and it left me with a positive impression of the VA. Instead of long waiting lists and being told "No" as I expected, I found a very caring and responsive environment where everyone tries to say "Yes." Although I get most of my care through TRICARE, it's nice to have another option for things that TRICARE does not cover.

Special Needs/ECHO Program

All TRICARE health plans include support for those with special needs. This includes applied behavioral analysis (ABA), skilled nursing, durable medical equipment (DME), etc. See **tricare.mil/CoveredServices/SpecialNeeds** for details.

The **Extended Care Health Option (ECHO)** provides supplemental services to **Active Duty Family Members (ADFMs) with qualifying mental or physical disabilities** and offers integrated services and supplies beyond those offered by TRICARE plans. To obtain these benefits, sponsors must sign up for the **Exceptional Family Member Program (EFMP)** through their military branch and register for ECHO with the regional contractor. ECHO coverage is <u>not</u> retroactive, so sign up as soon as possible.

Qualifying ADFMs must be enrolled in TRICARE Prime, Select, or U.S. Family Health Plan. ECHO benefits are available with a qualifying condition to:

- TRICARE-eligible ADFMs, including family members of National Guard and Reserve members ordered to active duty for more than 30 days.

- Family members who are eligible for continued coverage under the Transitional Assistance Management Program.

- Children or spouses of former service members who were victims of physical or emotional abuse.

- Family members of a deceased active duty sponsor while they are in transitional survivor status.

Conditions to qualify for ECHO coverage include, but are not limited to:

- Autism spectrum disorder
- Moderate or severe intellectual disability
- Serious physical disability
- Extraordinary physical or psychological condition of such complexity that the beneficiary is homebound
- Neuromuscular developmental condition or other condition in an infant or toddler (under age 3) that is expected to precede a diagnosis of moderate or severe intellectual disability or a serious physical disability
- Multiple disabilities, which may qualify if there are two or more disabilities affecting separate body systems

Children may remain eligible for ECHO benefits beyond the usual TRICARE eligibility age limit, provided all the following are true:

- The sponsor remains on active duty.
- The child is incapable of self-support because of a mental or physical incapacity that occurs prior to the loss of eligibility.
- The sponsor provides over 50 percent of the child's financial support.

For more information about EFMP, contact your service branch's EFMP representative. Learn more about ECHO benefits at **www.tricare.mil/Plans/SpecialPrograms/ECHO**

As of this writing, TRICARE is conducting an Autism Care Demonstration (ACD) to bring focused services to those on the autism spectrum. The scheduled end date is December 31, 2028, but it is not uncommon for such demonstrations to transition into core TRICARE benefits if they are found to be successful and cost-effective, or to phase out early if not.

One of the benefits under ACD is the assignment of an Autism Care Navigator (ACN) to your child. The role of the ACN is to coordinate care, monitor timelines and outcomes, and to connect you with other resources for your child's care. To learn about these resources and how to access them, visit **tricare.mil/Plans/SpecialPrograms**

Mental Health Coverage

TRICARE offers robust mental health coverage, including inpatient and outpatient care. In a mental health emergency for yourself or a loved one, call 911 or visit any emergency room without delay. There is also a nationwide suicide prevention and crisis hotline which you can reach by dialing 988 from any U.S. phone. Visit **988lifeline.org** for full details.

It is important that you visit an "authorized provider" for mental health care. A practitioner holding a certificate, rather than a medical license, is <u>not</u> an authorized provider, so their invoices will not be honored. Call your regional contractor to be sure. It is not uncommon for mental health providers to opt-out of federal health programs, freeing them from pricing constraints. This makes them non-authorized, and your TRICARE claim will not be honored.

For a complete description of mental health coverage, visit **tricare.mil/CoveredServices/Mental/Treatments**. Click "Covered Treatments" on that page to see what is and is not covered for mental health services and the conditions required for certain treatments. On the table of covered conditions, make sure to click "More" in the right-most column of that table to view any exclusions or pre-conditions for the treatment thar you are interested in.

TRICARE maintains a list of excluded mental health services. Because this list is subject to change, it is best to view the list online for the most current information. To view the list, visit **tricare.mil/CoveredServices/IsItCovered/ MentalHealthExclusions**

Depending on your plan and beneficiary status, there are different paths to obtaining care:

- **For a mental health emergency** when the patient is a threat to themselves or those around them, **seek emergency care without delay** at the nearest facility or by calling 911.

- **The 988 Suicide and Crisis Lifeline** is available around the clock to those facing mental health struggles, substance abuse, or thoughts of suicide. Dial 988 and press 1 if you are military, former military or calling about someone who is. Visit **988lifeline.org** for more information on this valuable service. It is available to all callers, even those with no military affiliation.

- Active duty, including activated Guard and Reservists, must seek care at their MTF if at all possible. Your PCM will coordinate any required referrals or authorization.

- Non-AD on Prime seeking **outpatient care** can see any network mental health provider without referral or authorization. If you visit a non-network provider without referral, you will be responsible for Point of Service fees (described under Prime in Chapter 7).

- Non-AD on Prime seeking **inpatient/residential mental health treatment** will need authorization and a referral from their regional contractor.

- Those in **USFHP** can seek outpatient care within their provider network without referral or preauthorization. Contact the plan provider for any inpatient/residential care, substance abuse treatment, or psychoanalysis.

- **Residential substance abuse treatment <u>always</u> requires pre-authorization from your regional contractor**, even if you already have a referral.

- **All other plans do NOT need referrals** for mental health outpatient care **<u>except for</u>** psychoanalysis or outpatient substance abuse therapy provided by a substance abuse rehabilitation facility. Inpatient care will require pre-authorization from your regional contractor.

Skilled Nursing Care

TRICARE covers skilled nursing either in a skilled nursing facility or at home with part-time, intermittent nursing visits. In both cases, pre-authorization is needed from your regional contractor. The care must be medically necessary, and there are certain prerequisites. For care in a skilled nursing facility, you must have been hospitalized for at least three days (not including the day of discharge), and care in the facility must begin within 30 days of discharge. Other rules apply.

Certain types of care that are **NOT** covered often get confused with skilled nursing. These include assisted living, convalescent homes, and long term care. Hospice care IS covered, but only within the United States and U.S. territories. It is not covered in international locations. Use the TRICARE "What's Covered" tool to learn more about these types of care.

Telemedicine/Telehealth

Telehealth services via secure video or audio-only visits are covered under TRICARE. This may include preventive health screenings, mental health care, and end-stage renal disease. Active duty service members must have a referral for telehealth.

Consultations must be medically necessary and appropriate to your condition. You must receive care from an authorized provider. For mental health care, see the earlier section for precautions on selecting a TRICARE-authorized provider and rules on obtaining referrals. Those guidelines apply equally to telemedicine.

If you are seeking telehealth services from an overseas location, telehealth must be legal in the country where you reside AND your provider must be licensed to practice both in your location and at their own. This makes international telehealth challenging to use when overseas.

Vaccinations

TRICARE covers age-appropriate vaccines and immunizations as recommended by the Centers for Disease Control (CDC). CDC guidance changes rather frequently, so check with your doctor or the CDC website for the current schedule of vaccines that apply to you and your family. Because vaccines and immunizations are considered preventive care, they should be provided at no cost to all beneficiaries under all TRICARE plans.

TRICARE will NOT cover vaccinations that are purely for the purpose of travel, except for travel under military orders for both the service member and accompanying family members. If you file such a claim, include a copy of the travel orders to validate the official requirement. If you will be traveling unofficially to a destination that requires a specific vaccine for entry, this will not be covered unless you can link it to a CDC recommendation.

Dental Coverage

Three dental plans listed below cover TRICARE beneficiaries. We are also listing a fourth option through the VA that is widely available to the veteran community.

- **Active Duty Dental Plan (ADDP)** is for active duty members as well as activated National Guard and Reservists. This covers the dental needs of military members and is always at no cost. Learn more at **tricare.mil/CoveredServices/Dental/ADDental/ADDP**.
- **TRICARE Dental Plan (TDP)** is for family members of active duty sponsors as well as non-activated Guard or Reserve members and their families. This is optional coverage, provided for a fee. To learn about costs,

benefits, and procedures for enrollment, visit
www.uccitdp.com/dtwdws/member/landing.xhtml

- **The Federal Employees Dental & Vision Insurance Program (FEDVIP)** covers military retirees and their dependents. FEDVIP is not part of TRICARE; it replaced the TRICARE Retiree Dental Program which ended in 2018. FEDVIP coverage is optional, for a fee. Visit **www.benefeds.com** for details.

- **Veterans and their families are eligible for the Veterans Affairs Dental Insurance Program (VADIP)** if the sponsor is in VA Health Care (see Chapter 10). VADIP is a collection of discounted commercial dental plans from providers like Delta Dental and MetLife. Learn more at **www.va.gov/health-care/about-va-health-benefits/dental-care/**

- **Survivors of sponsors who died on active duty** may be covered either by TRICARE Dental Survivor Benefit or FEDVIP. For surviving family members:

  - Spouses are eligible for TRICARE Dental Survivor Benefits for three years, beginning on the date of the sponsor's death.

  - Children are eligible until age 21, or age 23 if they are enrolled full time in an accredited college and meet other qualifying conditions.

  - Dental coverage during this period is 100 percent free to the family members.

  - Learn more at **tricare.mil/CoveredServices/ Dental RetireeSurvivorBenefit**

Adult children enrolled in TYA are <u>not</u> eligible for any dental programs under TRICARE.

Vision Care

TRICARE vision benefits depend on which plan you are in, your status (ADSM/ADFM/retiree) and the purchase of optional vision care through BENEFEDS/FEDVIP. Learn about TRICARE vision benefits at **tricare.mil/CoveredServices/Vision**. Information about vision plans for retirees and family members can be found at **www.benefeds.com**

- **Active Duty Service Members (ADSM)**
  - Full vision care at no cost.
  - Eye exams, glasses, or contacts provided through the MTF or through a network provider with referral.
  - Those in Prime Remote will need a referral.
  - An ADSM visiting a non-network provider **without** a referral may be responsible for the entire cost. This is one of the rare instances where free care for ADSM is not guaranteed. It is avoidable simply by getting a referral beforehand.

- **ADFM** (including family members of activated Guard or Reservists):
  - One routine eye exam per year regardless of TRICARE plan.
  - Glasses and contacts are not covered.
  - More complete vision coverage, including glasses, contacts, and discounted laser eye surgery, is available through the optional FEDVIP Program.

- **All other beneficiaries:**
  - One eye exam every two years in TRICARE Prime.
  - In USFHP, contact the provider for details.
  - In all other plans, routine eye exams are not covered.
  - Glasses and contacts are not included in any of these plans.

Children from age three until the sixth birthday can receive eye exams under their well-child benefits at no cost.

All TRICARE plans include ophthalmology services for the diagnosis and treatment of eye disorders. Ophthalmology covers, for example, the diagnosis and treatment of glaucoma and cataracts. Contact your regional contractor about coverage for such services under your TRICARE plan.

Retirees have two other options for obtaining vision care outside of their TRICARE plan:

- VA health care, discussed in Chapter 10
- The Naval Ophthalmic Readiness Activity (NORA)

NORA offers a service that provides no-cost eyeglasses to retirees by mail. You would have an eye exam conducted by your local optometrist and fill out the NORA prescription form to receive your glasses. For more information, see **www.med.navy.mil/Naval-Medical-Readiness-Logistics-Command/Naval-Ophthalmic-Readiness-Activity/**

Travel Expenses

Non-active duty beneficiaries in Prime or Prime Remote may be eligible for travel and lodging reimbursement under certain circumstances. To qualify, all the following must be true:

- Cannot be on active duty
- Must have a referral from the PCM
- Must be on Prime or Prime Remote
- The specialist must be more than 100 miles from the PCM's office.

If all four apply, you may qualify for the Prime Travel Benefit. Contact your MTF travel office to plan and coordinate your travel. Learn more at **tricare.mil/primetravel** or ask your regional contractor for more information.

Air Ambulance/Medical Evacuation

TRICARE offers **limited** coverage for medical evacuation or air ambulance. If you want more comprehensive or flexible coverage, you should research private commercial policies. For TRICARE air evacuation coverage:

- Transport must be **medically necessary** and regular land transport is not practicable.

- Air transport will take you to the **NEAREST hospital** that can safely provide the care you need. Most likely, this will <u>not</u> be a U.S. military facility.

- **TRICARE will not transport you to the U.S.** unless that is the nearest place for the type of care you need. Transport to the U.S. is called **"repatriation"** and can be purchased commercially.

- For ADSM/ADFM enrollees in Prime or Prime Remote, ISOS can coordinate for a cashless transaction. All others must pay for the transport upfront and then submit a claim for reimbursement. This can be quite expensive, with the risk of not being reimbursed.

- If it is determined that the transport was not medically necessary, **your claim may be denied.**

As you can see, TRICARE coverage has significant risks and limitations. If air evacuation coverage is important to you, consider purchasing a commercial policy. Coverage can be purchased on a yearly basis or for shorter terms, with or without its own medical coverage.

Many commercial packages:

- Guarantee your return to the U.S. to continue your medical care.
- Do not require a finding of medical necessity.
- Require little or no upfront funds from you, other than your prepaid premium.

Join our Facebook group *"TRICARE Around the World"* to discuss this further and to get recommendations from other members. You can learn more about medical transport at **tricare.mil/CoveredServices/IsItCovered/AirEvacuation**

Expert Tip: The terms "air ambulance" or "air evacuation" also may be called "medical evacuation" or "repatriation." The term "repatriation" can refer either to the medical transport of a patient or the return of remains after death. Some policies will include medical coverage while others are for transport only. Clarify these terms with the insurer when shopping for policies.

Expert Tip: If you live in a rural area within the United States, far from any advanced trauma care, consider contacting "life flight" services in your area. You may be able to sign up for an annual contract that covers your transport to emergency/trauma care if needed. Contact your sheriff's department to find out which air ambulance providers are used in your area. If there are several, you might have to sign up for each one, with an annual fee. This can save precious hours and large fees if you ever are airlifted for emergency care.

TRICARE on Cruise Ships

You might be surprised to learn that TRICARE can be used on cruise ships. It works just the same as any other setting: Get the medical care you need and pay the cruise line. **Be sure to get an <u>itemized</u> receipt and medical report for your claim.** If you will be hospitalized, notify your regional contractor at the first opportunity.

If you have purchased travel insurance that offers medical coverage, then TRICARE becomes second payer. File your claim first with the travel policy. Once you receive the Explanation of Benefits (EOB), submit a claim to TRICARE for any unpaid costs and attach the EOB to your claim.

Three major precautions apply:

- TRICARE has a reimbursement limit for all types of care. Medical fees at sea are extraordinarily high, so it is possible to exceed TRICARE cost limits onboard a ship. Any excess will come out of your pocket.

- The ship's location can impact your costs. If the ship is in a U.S. port or U.S. territorial waters, and you are on TFL, then Medicare will work. Outside U.S. territorial waters, you cannot use Medicare. Ask the cruise operator for the precise location so you can anticipate your costs.

- For those in a TRICARE Prime plan, obtaining routine care without a referral is Point of Service care, with higher deductibles and copayments. For a description of the POS option, see Chapter 7 under TRICARE Prime.

Expert Tip: If you become sick on a cruise, consider obtaining care ashore rather than onboard. Medical fees aboard ship may exceed TRICARE reimbursement limits while care ashore is likely to be far cheaper. You will have to judge whether a delay in treatment is advisable and if the quality of care at the port-of-call meets your standards. If possible, contact the MHS Nurse Advice Line for advice. See Chapter 14 for more information about the Nurse Advice Line.

Real Life Story: CPAP with TRICARE

I have twice conducted a sleep study and obtained a CPAP (Continuous Positive Airway Pressure) machine using my TRICARE benefits. The first, in 2015, was at Tripler Army Medical Center in Hawaii as a retiree on Prime. The second, in 2020, was at a private hospital in Bangkok, Thailand, using TRICARE Overseas Select.

There are two ways a sleep study can be done:

- In a specially equipped hospital room where the patient's breathing, heartbeat, blood oxygen level, snoring, and body movements are monitored through the night. This is what I had done in Thailand.

- A home-based study with equipment provided by your doctor. This is what I did in Hawaii as the in-hospital sleep study is for active duty members only.

If you are offered an at-home sleep study, consider asking for a referral to a civilian facility for the more thorough in-hospital method. This request may or may not be granted. In 2015, I was not knowledgeable enough to make that request, so I did the home test which is much less thorough.

For my sleep study in Thailand, I slept the first half of the night without a CPAP to create a baseline of my condition. Then I was awakened and fitted with a mask to assess how well my symptoms were alleviated by the CPAP. The overnight stay is not considered to be inpatient care because you are not admitted for treatment; your TRICARE copayment will be calculated as specialty care, not inpatient care.

With TRICARE Prime in Hawaii, I was not given a choice of which CPAP device I got. Tripler sent me to a local supplier who had a CPAP ready for me. It was preset to the parameters my doctor had prescribed, and the vendor provided a few hurried minutes of instruction on a warehouse loading dock. For five years, I hoped that the settings were good because I didn't know how to verify or change them.

When I got my second CPAP in Thailand, TRICARE Overseas assured me that I could buy from any vendor and then submit a claim. I could have ordered online from the States but chose to buy from a supplier in Bangkok. One consideration is that while TRICARE covers the cost of shipping, they do NOT reimburse customs/import fees. Import fees of medical devices are quite steep in Thailand, so shipping from the States would have cost me a lot out of pocket. By buying locally, TRICARE Select reimbursed 75 percent of the cost. At the time, it was the largest claim I had ever submitted, and it was a great relief to see that the reimbursement process worked as advertised.

Unlike my experience in Hawaii, the vendor representative in Thailand came to my home, set up the machine, and provided hands-on instruction. She let me borrow a CPAP for two nights to make sure that it was satisfactory. Once I made the purchase decision, she came back to finalize the paperwork and link the CPAP to my iPhone. Customer service was vastly superior to what I had experienced in the States.

With TRICARE Prime, I did not own the machine; I leased it for a small payment each month. For the first few months, I was monitored by my PCM to ensure that I was using the device each night; TRICARE won't want to pay for the monthly lease if you are not using the machine regularly. With TRICARE Select, I own the machine because I bought it outright. There are no monthly fees and no monitoring. There is a cost-share for hoses and masks, so I ordered these through VA Health Care instead, which has no out-of-pocket cost to me. Because of the ability to choose the machine I wanted, plus the in-hospital sleep study and excellent customer support, I found my experience with TRICARE Select in Thailand to be far superior to what I went through with TRICARE Prime in the States. Your outcome may be different.

5
Finding A Provider

ONE OF THE THINGS THAT MEMBERS FIND MOST CONFUSING about TRICARE is locating health care providers whether in the States, living abroad, or when traveling. Questions we frequently hear are: *Who can I see, when can I see them, and how do I find them?* Finding answers is easier than you might think.

This chapter describes the different types of providers and assistance available to you worldwide. Visit this page **www.tricare.mil/GettingCare/GettingCareSpecialScenarios** for a TRICARE roadmap to finding doctors in a variety of situations. If the link no longer works, just search the TRICARE website for the word "traveling."

Authorized Providers

The TRICARE website says that you must see "TRICARE-authorized providers." How do you figure out who these providers are? Is there a list somewhere? A search engine?

- **Within the U.S.,** one way to locate providers is to click "Find a Doctor" on the TRICARE site. This search tool can find providers by ZIP Code in any number of medical specialties. Experience has shown that the search tool doesn't always work well, so we have come to rely on other strategies as explained in the next section.

- **Outside the U.S.,** the term "authorized" is not used in the same way. In TRICARE's words, you may visit **any provider who is *"licensed by a state, accredited by a national organization, or meets other standards of the medical community."*** In other words, if your overseas provider holds a medical license

where they practice, they are an "authorized provider."
There is no list.

This revelation is game-changing! This one simple rule is what compelled me to start a Facebook group and share my findings with the world. Once you understand that you can visit virtually <u>any</u> licensed international hospital, clinic, or doctor, the use of TRICARE globally suddenly becomes so much easier.

Naturally, there are exclusions and exceptions. For instance, members of Prime plans need referrals or pre-authorization for routine care to avoid high fees. The Philippines has its own unique search engine for finding providers (see Chapter 9). You might find it advantageous to seek out network providers – which can be found in many cities around the world – to reduce your costs. But overall, TRICARE is largely demystified once you understand how broadly accessible it is wherever you go.

Expert Tip: In a medical emergency, you can go to almost any Emergency Room regardless of your TRICARE plan. However, on rare occasions, members of our Facebook group have encountered NON-authorized ERs in the States. These non-authorized providers are stand-alone emergency rooms, not physically attached to a hospital. If you encounter a standalone ER, be aware that they might not be TRICARE-authorized, and your medical expenses there may not be reimbursed. The best plan is to research in advance of a medical need.

Choosing a PCM or Primary Doctor

If you are in a TRICARE Prime plan, you will be assigned a Primary Care Manager (PCM) during your enrollment process. Your PCM is the doctor or other health care professional you will see for most non-emergency care. Your PCM may be at an MTF or a civilian facility, but all your care will be handled within the TRICARE network, making health management much simpler.

Be careful during enrollment – just because you are assigned to a PCM does not mean that they are available! People sometimes find that their assigned PCM has left the network or is not accepting new patients. Call the PCM to be sure. If there are any issues, you can request a change of PCM.

With non-Prime plans, you will not have a PCM. You are empowered to choose your primary doctor and specialists and make many healthcare decisions on your own. Though not required by TRICARE, it is prudent to choose a primary doctor to give you continuity of care and to aid in prescription renewals or create referrals when required by a specialty clinic. Each family member can choose their own primary doctor.

To find doctors when our family moved to Hawaii, we worked the problem in reverse. We chose a local hospital that offered comprehensive services including a 24-hour emergency room. We confirmed that they were in-network for Select and then asked how to find a family doctor for our routine needs. The hospital referred us to their online list of affiliated doctors, told us to pick one and call to see if they were accepting new patients. The online directory allowed us to easily search. Most doctors have their own practice in town, near our home, making routine visits quite convenient. Because these doctors are affiliated with a network hospital, all the specialists they refer us to are also in network, so the plan works seamlessly.

Overseas, it will be somewhat different. You are not going to find a vast array of network providers to meet all your needs. You may be lucky to find any in-network provider at all. In this case, find a hospital or clinic that you like, preferably one that accepts credit cards since many parts of the world are cash-only for medical care. Our criteria for finding overseas providers are: High-quality care, speaks English, accepts credit cards. This makes getting care overseas quite easy and convenient. After seeing your overseas provider, pay the bill in full, then submit a claim for reimbursement. Chapters 12 and 13 cover this in detail.

Search Strategies

How do you find TRICARE authorized providers? You can use the TRICARE Provider Finder tool, but this does not always work well. The tool can yield false positives (listing someone in-network when they are not) or false negatives (telling you that no provider is available when, in fact, they are). You need other ways to research.

Besides the search tool, you may inquire at the nearest MTF, ask within the local military community, talk to your regional contractor or the Nurse Advice Line, post in our Facebook group, or call any provider to ask if they are in-network. None of these are foolproof; you just have to be diligent in your search.

Outside the U.S., finding a network provider can be even more challenging. There may not be any in your area, or they might be in-network for some situations (e.g., inpatient care or active duty only) but not for others. The TRICARE Overseas call centers are often unable to tell you who is in-network, and even the hospital itself might not be sure. From discussions in our Facebook group, we are aware of network providers in Thailand, Germany, Italy, France, UK, South Korea, Panama and Japan. There are bound to be some in other countries as well, if you can find them. There is no coherent or consistent list to be found. Overseas, you should be prepared to deal with non-network providers, filing claims for reimbursement. Under that assumption, using TRICARE globally is quite easy and responsive.

Network Providers

When possible, you should use TRICARE network providers. This is advantageous for several reasons:

- Stateside, network providers are relatively plentiful, so there is a good chance that one is nearby.

- In most cases, the in-network copayment will be cheaper than a non-network cost-share. For smaller bills, this can be inverted. See our **Real Life Story** at the end of this section to learn how this can happen.

- After you pay the deductible and copayment, the provider will send the remaining portion of the bill to the regional contractor for payment. This means you pay less money upfront and will not have to submit a claim.

If you are in one of the TRICARE Prime options, your PCM may refer you to network specialists as needed. If your PCM refers you to a non-network provider, you will be charged only the network copay because you have a referral. If you are in Prime and see a specialist without a referral – even a network provider – this is called Point of Service (POS) and it will be very expensive for you. Learn more about POS in Chapter 7 under TRICARE Prime.

With non-Prime plans, you can visit network or non-network providers at your discretion. With a network provider, your copayment will be a flat fee. With non-network, your cost-share is a percentage of the bill. For less expensive visits, a network provider could cost more than a non-network provider. See the Real Life Story below about this.

In the Philippines, "Preferred" providers are roughly equivalent to network providers. They are found in the major urban areas of Metro Manila, Subic, and Clark/Angeles City. See Chapter 9 for more information about finding providers in the Philippines.

Real Life Story: Saving Money with a Non-Network Provider

How can a non-network provider end up cheaper than a network one? We once went to an emergency room in Bangkok. The bill was $120, and we expected our share to be 25 percent of that, just $30. Once the claim was settled, however, our cost was $50. When I asked why, ISOS said it was because we had gone to a network hospital, and the network copayment was a flat $50. If we had gone to a non-network provider, we would have had a 25 percent cost-share, or $30.

Fortunately, this was an inexpensive mistake costing us just an extra $20, but it was a great learning experience. This "inverted" price structure can happen with smaller bills where a non-network 25 percent cost-share may be cheaper than a network flat rate copayment. This often holds true for Physical Therapy or Occupational Therapy where individual sessions are relatively inexpensive. In these cases, group members have found it cheaper to visit non-network therapists. The math will change each year as the cost of copayments increase.

Non-Network Providers

Non-network providers:

- Have no formal agreement with TRICARE.
- Are unlikely to file claims for you.
- Will require full payment from you, after which you will submit a claim for reimbursement.

Within the category of non-network providers, there are **Participating** and **Non-Participating providers**. Participating providers agree to accept the TRICARE allowable charge as full payment, so you won't be stuck with excess fees that are not covered by TRICARE. Non-participating providers have no such agreement, so it is possible that their fees can exceed TRICARE's allowable reimbursement limits. You would not be reimbursed for the excess fees.

Outside the U.S., the vast majority of providers are non-network. You pay the bill at discharge and submit a claim at your earliest convenience. Once you practice this skill a few times, you can reasonably expect to get your reimbursement in just a few weeks. See Chapters 12 and 13 for details of filing claims.

Emergency Care

If you are in the midst of a medical emergency and trying to figure out what to do – **_STOP!_** Go to the nearest emergency room or call an ambulance. Emergency care is covered under **all** TRICARE plans worldwide. If you are unsure if your situation qualifies as an emergency, contact the MHS Nurse Advice Line at **mhsnurseadviceline.com**; they will advise you what to do. **Active duty members should try to seek care at an MTF if feasible.** If, however, this will delay emergency care, then go to the nearest civilian ER or call an ambulance.

If your concern is about how to pay a potentially large bill for emergency care, call your TRICARE regional contractor once the crisis has been dealt with; they may be able to arrange direct payment to the hospital. Phone numbers for TRICARE regional call centers are listed under "Global Resources" in Chapter 14. If you are overseas, the cost of emergency care is likely to be far less than in the United States—sometimes just $100 or so.

Emergency care – as well as medically-necessary ambulance transport – is covered by TRICARE, period! Get the care you need and sort out the billing later. Please read the Expert Tip earlier in this chapter (under "Authorized Providers") to find one precaution when choosing an emergency room for your care.

Urgent Care Clinics

Urgent Care is medical care needed for a non-emergency illness or injury that:

- Is not a threat to life, limb, or eyesight.
- Needs attention before it becomes a serious risk to health.
- Should receive attention within 24 hours to avoid further risk or complications.

The Ultimate Guide to TRICARE

Examples may include conditions like a sprained ankle, infection, minor cuts or burns, or fever. **If you are unsure whether urgent care is warranted, contact the MHS Nurse Advice Line to talk with a registered nurse.**

The rules governing access to urgent care depend largely on the status of the patient:

- An ADSM who lives in a Prime Service Area should visit an MTF for urgent care or call the MHS Nurse Advice Line for assistance.

- An ADSM in Prime Remote can visit any TRICARE-authorized clinic without referral.

- Retirees, their family members, and ADFMs do not need a referral. Those in Prime may incur POS fees if they visit a non-network facility without prior authorization.

- Beneficiaries in USFHP should consult their provider's website for guidance.

- Remember: TRICARE Plus and Direct Care Only (DCO) will **not** reimburse care from civilian providers, which includes Urgent Care Clinics.

Visit **tricare.mil/CoveredServices/IsItCovered/UrgentCare** for further details.

Nurse Advice Line

One of the most useful resources is the Military Health System (MHS) Nurse Advice Line. This free service gives you 24/7 access to very knowledgeable nurses who work at MHS, the parent organization of TRICARE. They are trained in assessing symptoms and health-related issues, and you also can ask for a pediatric nurse if calling about a child. They understand your TRICARE benefits in depth and can direct you to the most appropriate health resources in your community. If you are unsure whether your health issue is covered by TRICARE or who to see for medical care, the Nurse Advice Line can help.

Visit **mhsnurseadviceline.com** or call 1-800-TRICARE (874-2273). There are some tricks to accessing the help line from overseas which are explained in Chapter 14 in the section titled "MHS Nurse Advice Line."

Direct Billing Providers

A common misperception is to confuse network providers with those who direct bill. This misunderstanding might be costing you money. Direct-billing providers – even if they are non-network – will charge you your deductible and copayment and then bill TRICARE for the rest. To calculate this amount, they must contact your regional contractor to determine whether you have satisfied your deductible for the year and find out your cost-share. If you have reached your catastrophic cap for the year, you may not have to pay anything at all.

It is difficult to know which providers will direct bill since TRICARE does not keep a list, and providers can change their mind about it. Direct-bill providers do not need permission from TRICARE to bill directly; it is simply a business decision on their part, and you may be able to persuade them to try. Your best source of information about this is our Facebook group and from the military expats in your area.

Real Life Story: Direct Billing in Thailand

I was fortunate enough to find a direct-billing hospital for cataract surgery in Pattaya, Thailand in 2020. The procedure cost around $10,000, but my family had nearly reached our catastrophic cap for the year. The insurance office of the Thai hospital called the TRICARE Overseas regional office in Singapore, confirmed that the procedure was covered, and calculated my copayment up to the cap, so that I ended up paying just a few hundred dollars. Much of my payment was for an upgrade to my lens implant which was not covered by TRICARE. The rest of the bill was sent to TRICARE, and I did not have to deal with billing or claims.

Expert Tip: If you are facing expensive inpatient care, ask your hospital if they would be willing to bill TRICARE directly. Larger hospitals are skilled in dealing with insurance carriers from all over the world. If they agree to bill TRICARE directly, they will call your regional contractor to confirm your coverage. You will pay only your deductible and cost-share, and the remaining bill will be sent to TRICARE. If you have reached your catastrophic cap, you may have no out-of-pocket costs at all!

Point of Service Option

Point of Service (POS) is an option for enrollees in any Prime plan (Prime, Prime Remote, or TYA-Prime) to receive routine (non-emergency) care without a referral.

With the POS option, members can expect:

- A higher deductible than normal.
- A 50 percent copay after meeting the POS deductible.
- More stringent limits on allowable costs, which may increase the member's copay if the limit is exceeded.

The most important financial impact is that **POS fees do not count towards your annual catastrophic cap.** This means that there is **NO LIMIT** on how much you might have to pay. Use POS judiciously or – better yet – not at all.

POS fees do not apply to:

- ADSM, for whom care is always free.
- Anyone on a non-Prime plan.
- A Prime member who has a referral from their PCM.
- Emergency care and, in most cases, urgent care. Read the Expert Tip under the Chapter 5 section on Authorized Providers for a precaution on choosing an emergency room.

The POS option is discussed further in Chapter 7 in the section about TRICARE Prime.

Overseas Residents Visiting the USA

If you live overseas and are planning to visit the U.S., there are some things that you should know beforehand. Members of Prime or Prime Remote should obtain any routine care <u>before</u> travels begin, including prescription refills. For routine care while traveling, Prime members will need a referral from your PCM. This is not always granted.

Those on Overseas Select may visit any authorized provider in the U.S. for routine, urgent or emergency care, just as they would in their overseas location. Remember that, in the States, network providers are far more plentiful than overseas, meaning your out-of-pocket costs can be less.

Members in TRICARE for Life (TFL) have an added advantage when visiting the States because Medicare starts working as soon as they enter the country. No referral is needed. As long as you visit a Medicare provider, your Medicare cost-shares are covered by TFL, and you pay nothing. This is why many overseas members in TFL periodically return to the States to catch up on expensive medical care. This also gives you a chance to renew prescriptions from a U.S. doctor, which Express Scripts can then refill by mail if you have access to an APO or FPO address abroad (except in Germany, which does not allow medications by mail).

U.S. Residents Traveling Abroad

Let's look at the opposite situation: What if you are enrolled in a stateside plan and need care while traveling overseas? If this happens to you, call an ambulance, go to an emergency room or visit any licensed health care provider without delay. **For those in a Prime plan, notify TRICARE Overseas by phone within 24 hours of obtaining emergency care or being**

admitted as an inpatient. ISOS might be able to arrange bill payment for Prime members, reducing your need for cash. This notification is not needed if you are in TRICARE Select or TFL, and there is NEVER a requirement to call in advance or get pre-approval for emergency care.

If you are unsure as to what warrants urgent or emergency care, call the MHS Nurse Advice Line. A friendly, informed nurse will answer all your TRICARE questions and can advise you where to go for care. This line is open 24/7/365. See Chapter 14 for tips on using the Nurse Advice Line.

Active duty members should seek treatment at an MTF when traveling overseas, if possible, but don't let this delay necessary emergency care. In emergencies, seek the nearest care. For urgent care, you should not have to drive more than 30 minutes. There will be no cost to ADSMs, even if you must initially pay out of pocket. After submitting a claim, you will be fully reimbursed.

6
TRICARE Costs

WHEN ASSESSING THE COST of TRICARE coverage, people often focus on the monthly fees and copayments. While these are important, fees and copayments are not the only cost element and perhaps not even the most significant. It is essential that beneficiaries understand all aspects of cost so that they can best protect their family. This chapter will explain all components of TRICARE costs and their significance so you can choose the plan that best meets your needs.

Cost Definitions

To fully understand the cost of your health plan, you need to understand certain basic terms. Confusion about fees, deductibles, copayments, and catastrophic cap can lead people to make bad decisions about enrollment. We even have seen members reject TRICARE entirely because they misunderstand catastrophic cap or other important terms. This is an expensive and unnecessary mistake. The following definitions are the building blocks to understanding your costs.

Fee or premium: This is the amount you pay monthly, quarterly, or annually to enroll in your plan. It can be paid from retiree pay, automated bank transfer, or with a credit card. Fee and premium are not exactly the same.

- **Fee-based plans are taxpayer-subsidized.** The actual cost of medical care is largely borne by taxpayers, making these plans quite affordable for enrolled members. Examples of fee-based plans include Prime and Select.

- **Premium-based plans are NOT taxpayer-subsidized.** The cost of medical care under these plans is borne by the plan enrollees, without relying on tax dollars. For this reason, the cost of premium-based plans is much higher than fee-based plans. Such plans include TRICARE Young Adult and TRICARE Reserve Select.

Copayment or cost-share: This is your share of the medical expense when you obtain care. The amount varies by which plan you are in, the status of your sponsor, and the type of care that you receive. The TRICARE Cost Tool, explained later in this chapter, will tell you exactly what your copayment or cost-share will be in any particular situation.

- **Cost-share** is a percentage of the bill that you would pay, such as a 25 percent cost-share that a retiree pays for seeing a non-network provider under TRICARE Select.

- **Copayment** is a fixed dollar amount that you are billed, such as a $50 flat fee for seeing certain specialists.

Deductible: Deductible is an amount that you must pay out of pocket each year before your TRICARE benefits kick in. Not all plans have a deductible; consequently, benefits start from the very first dollar spent. For plans with a deductible, there is both an individual deductible and a family deductible.

- Once an individual meets their deductible, TRICARE begins covering a share of that person's health costs for the rest of the year.

- The family deductible is met once two family members have met their individual deductibles. At that point, no other family members will have to satisfy an individual deductible, and the entire family will have their expenses covered in accordance with their plan. This is of value for families of three or more, since only two family members have to meet a deductible.

- The deductible is assessed only once per year. Once met, there are no more deductibles for the remainder of the calendar year. Some people mistakenly believe that a deductible is assessed for each visit, all year long. This is not true! You likely will satisfy your deductible after just one or two medical visits.

Deductibles vary, depending on which plan you are in and the type of provider you visit.

- **Prime plans have no deductible,** so your benefits start from your very first medical bill. You will pay only your normal cost-share, if any.

- **With non-Prime plans,** if you are seeing a **network provider,** their billing office should be able to determine whether or not you have met your deductible for the year. If you have not, then your deductible amount will be payable by you to the provider. If your deductible has been met, you will be billed only for your normal copayment. If you are incorrectly billed your deductible twice, such as two claims in process at the same time, the overpayment will be refunded to you by either the provider or your regional contractor.

- **Non-network providers** generally do not check whether or not you have met your deductible. You pay the bill in full and submit a claim. Your reimbursement will withhold the deductible amount from your first claim. Some people fail to submit that first claim because they know the deductible will be withheld, giving them little or no reimbursement. The truth is that you cannot meet the deductible until you file a claim; this is a necessary step towards getting benefits in any given year. <u>Please commit to filing that **first** claim</u> each year so that your benefits can begin!

Catastrophic cap: This is the most a family will pay out of pocket in a calendar year for covered care. Once the cap has been met, all further covered care is paid 100 percent by TRICARE with no copayments.

- Fees, deductibles, cost-shares, and copayments all count towards your cap. These add up until your cap is reached. While fees count towards the cap, premiums do not. Medicare fees also do not count, for those on TRICARE for Life.

- The catastrophic cap is per family, not per person. Once a family meets its cap for the year, then the entire family will have no more copayments, cost-shares, or fees for the rest of the year.

- If family members are in different plans, some may have lower caps than others. This means that some family members might become 100 percent covered earlier in the year, and other members a bit later on.

- The catastrophic cap may well be the least understood part of the TRICARE cost structure, and yet it is perhaps the most valuable. With a low cap in place, the worst case for your medical expenses in any given year may be just a few thousand dollars. If even this amount is financially painful, you might consider buying a TRICARE supplement to cover your copayments until your cap is reached. Supplement plans are discussed in Chapter 1.

Some people have a fundamental misunderstanding of the cap. They may be under the impression that it is the maximum amount that TRICARE will pay over the course of a year, so they believe their benefits are worth only a few thousand dollars. This mistaken belief is just plain wrong! The cap is the most that a *family* will pay, shielding them from financial ruin if they are facing catastrophic medical costs in a given year.

This is the sequence of how cost is shared between patient and TRICARE each year. <u>Please note that not all members or plans have deductibles or copayments</u>.

1. First, you sign up for a plan and start paying fees or premiums.

2. With the first medical bill each year, you pay out of pocket until the deductible is met. If your plan has no deductible, then your benefits start from the very first dollar billed.

3. One the deductible has been satisfied, then cost sharing begins. The member will pay some of the cost (copayment or cost-share) and TRICARE pays the remainder.

4. Once out-of-pocket costs for the entire family add up to the catastrophic cap, you will have no more costs for the year. TRICARE pays for all covered care for the rest of the year. Even your monthly fees should stop and will resume the following calendar year. Regrettably, this does not apply to premiums. If you pre-paid fees for the entire year, none of that will be refunded, but all the fees paid WILL count towards satisfying your cap.

Sponsor Group: Date of sponsor's initial military service determines whether the sponsor and their family members are in Group A or B. The sponsor group affects the cost of your plan.

- Group A are those sponsors whose military service began prior to January 1, 2018.

- Group B are those for whom military service began on or after January 1, 2018.

Consumer Protections

As of this writing, there are two consumer protections in place to protect against excessive medical billing within the United States: The No Surprise Act, and the Balance Billing Act.

The No Surprise Act does not apply to TRICARE, Medicare, Medicaid, VA Health Care, or Indian Health Services. These programs have other protections that meet or exceed the No Surprise Act. The law protects patients from unexpected medical bills – or "surprise billing" – by limiting the amount that patients can be charged by **non-providers** at an **in-network** facility during an emergency or some non-emergency situations. It requires that patients be notified when someone on their care team is out-of-network and limits their cost to normal in-network cost-shares.

Balance billing is the practice of billing a beneficiary the difference between the TRICARE allowed amount and the billed charges on a claim. Participating providers are prohibited from charging above TRICARE allowed amounts. Non-participating providers may bill 115 percent of the allowed charge. If you receive a bill that you believe exceeds this, you can call the provider or wait for your EOB to arrive and share that with the provider. The EOB shows the amount that you should pay. Most providers will adjust their billing upon request once they receive the EOB. If not, call your regional contractor.

The TRICARE Cost Tool

Until January 2025, the TRICARE website hosted a wonderful resource called the Cost Compare Tool. The tool would create a tailored spreadsheet for your family showing fees, deductibles, copayments, annual cap, and so forth. Better yet, you could compare two plans side-by-side to see which is the most advantageous for you. The tool was simple, easy-to-use, detailed and accurate.

Regrettably, this tool vanished when the new TRICARE contract was launched in 2025. It has been replaced by a series of PDFs that explain your costs. The information seems to be equally accurate, but not as intuitive as the older tool, and does not allow you to compare two plans side-by-side.

In the hope that this tool will one day be restored to the website, we are sharing instructions for the Cost Compare Tool. If you don't see the tool online, then click the Cost button as shown below and follow instructions to find the cost spreadsheet for your family. Either method should create an accurate description of your costs.

The Cost Compare Tool works best on a computer or tablet, not a smartphone.

1. Visit the TRICARE homepage at **www.tricare.mil**

2. At the top, click "Cost".

3. On the Cost page, click "TRICARE Compare Cost Tool".

4. The next page will ask a series of questions such as sponsor status (active duty, retired, etc.), Sponsor Group (A or B), and so forth. Answer each question one by one.

   a. For USFHP and TRICARE Prime Remote, select Prime from the pull-down menu.

   b. If the original uniformed sponsor is deceased, select "Survivor" as the sponsor status.

   c. If you are an unremarried spouse on CHCBP, choose "Retired", regardless of sponsor status.

5. A complete table of costs is now presented. Use the buttons above the table to either download in spreadsheet form or to print/save as a PDF.

6. **To compare two different plans:** Without clearing the current results, look above your cost table and answer the questions again, this time selecting a different TRICARE plan. This will add a column to your table with costs for the second plan right next to the first one.

If the Cost Compare Tool is no longer available, simply scroll down the Cost page until you see your plan and status (such as "TRICARE Select, Active Duty Family Member") and click to view your costs.

Other Cost Factors

Other factors come into play that may affect your cost. These are some of the most common.

Active Duty Service Members (ADSM): For ADSM, medical costs should always be zero. If you do have to pay out-of-pocket costs for any reason, save your receipts and the medical report, and submit a claim to your regional contractor for full reimbursement. You are also required to notify your PCM at your earliest opportunity for outside care received.

Medicare/TRICARE for Life (TFL): The cost of using TFL depends on whether the member is within the United States or overseas. Please see Chapter 8 for full details of Medicare and TFL.

- **Inside the U.S. and territories,** Medicare is the first payer, and TFL covers deductibles and copayments. The member's final cost is normally zero.
- **Internationally,** Medicare cannot be used. TFL is first payer, and the member will have copayments or cost shares until the catastrophic cap is met.

Point of Service (POS) option for TRICARE Prime: The Point of Service option is a way for non-AD members on TRICARE Prime to get routine care without a referral. We do not recommend using this approach, however, because your copayments are 50 percent of the total charges, plus you will have a special deductible. Worse yet, none of the costs incurred under POS will count towards your catastrophic cap, so there is no limit on how much you might have to pay. Use this option with extreme caution or not at all. You can learn more about the Prime POS Option at **tricare.mil/Costs/POS**

Dental Costs

There are three different dental plans available to TRICARE beneficiaries, depending on their status.

- The **Active Duty Dental Program (ADDP)** is for ADSM who are not located near a military dental facility. It is not available to family members. Dental services are 100 percent free. Visit **secure.addp-ucci.com/adsm** for more information.

- The **TRICARE Dental Plan (TDP)** is for ADFM plus certain non-activated reservists and their families. It is optional coverage, so those who do not enroll will not have any dental coverage through TRICARE. Cost varies depending on the sponsor's military status. Visit **tricare.mil/Costs/DentalCosts/TDP/Premiums** to find current costs.

- Retiree dental plans can be purchased through FEDVIP, which is separate from TRICARE. There are a variety of plans offered by different contractors, and costs vary per plan. Each plan has a downloadable PDF with a full table of costs and benefits. Visit **www.benefeds.com** for further details.

Unlike TRICARE, it is required that the sponsor enroll in dental in order to enroll any additional family members. If the sponsor is already using VA for dental, this is an additional cost that you will have to consider. The dental plans are broadly grouped into "High" and "Standard" categories. High plans give more generous coverage but with correspondingly higher monthly premiums. Cost varies by ZIP code, so there is no "one size fits all." Balance the needs of your family versus the cost of the plan to see what is best for you. Other alternatives include:

- Use employer-provided dental coverage which is often much cheaper than FEDVIP plans.

- Find a local dentist who offers annual coverage plans for your family at a discount.

- Self-insure, which means bear the risk of paying for dental care out-of-pocket, without any coverage at all. Many dental offices offer a discount if you do not have insurance, and a further discount if you pay cash.

If you live overseas, pay particular attention to plan benefits when using non-network providers. Many FEDVIP plans have little value internationally where the cost of dental care is much lower than in the USA.

Vision Costs

Vision care is free for active duty members and normally will be provided at an MTF. For those on Prime Remote, call to determine your source of vision care.

Retirees families and ADFM have access to vision care through FEDVIP at **www.benefeds.com.** Follow the online questionnaire to determine eligibility. A variety of commercial plans are available, and each has a downloadable brochure which explains benefits and costs. ADFM must be in a TRICARE plan to enroll in a FEDVIP vision plan. FEDVIP is not part of TRICARE and is billed separately.

7
TRICARE Plans

THIS CHAPTER PROVIDES A SUMMARY of each TRICARE plan. To find complete descriptions on the **tricare.mil** site, select "Health Plans" from the Plans & Eligibility menu.

Each TRICARE plan is considered either **managed or non-managed care**. They are also designated as either **premium-based or fee-based**. Knowing the designation of your plan will help you to better understand its cost structure and how to use your benefits.

- **Managed care plans** are TRICARE Prime, Prime Remote, TRICARE Young Adult (Prime), and U.S. Family Health Plan (USFHP). With managed care, you are assigned a Primary Care Manager (PCM) who is usually your first stop, other than emergency or urgent care. Your PCM will refer you to specialists as needed, and your regional contractor will manage and approve the referral. If you get specialty care without an approved referral, you will incur significantly higher costs.

- **Non-managed care plans**, also called **self-directed care**, consist of all plans not listed above. Under non-managed care, you do not have a PCM. You can choose your own providers and make appointments without a referral. Fees and payment terms vary depending on your plan and whether you see a network or a non-network provider. It is common for beneficiaries to choose a family doctor whom they will see regularly, but this is not a requirement under self-directed care.

- **Fee-based plans** are government-subsidized and are generally quite affordable. The amount of the fee is set by legislation. Prime and Select are examples of fee-based plans. Monthly fees and deductibles count towards the family's catastrophic cap. ADSM and ADFM are exempt from fees, as are some other beneficiaries.

- **Premium-based plans** are not government-subsidized. The full cost of insurance is borne by enrollees in these plans. Cost may rival that of commercial plans on the open market but still may be the most affordable option. If premium-based is your only option, it would be wise to shop in the Affordable Care Act (ACA) marketplace to make sure TRICARE is your best alternative. Compare not just the premium but also the deductible, copayment, and catastrophic cap. Examples of premium-based plans are TRICARE Young Adult and TRICARE Retired Reserve. Monthly premiums do **not** count towards a family's annual catastrophic cap.

In choosing a TRICARE plan, members often focus on cost, but **just as important is whether you would feel more comfortable in a managed or non-managed care setting.** Would you prefer seeing a PCM who can make referrals for you, or would you find it easier to make your own health care arrangements? Those on Prime might get most of their care at a Military Treatment Facility (MTF), which is a more comfortable and familiar setting to many. Those transitioning from military service often default to TRICARE Prime because it's what they are used to from their military days.

The remainder of this chapter describes each of the TRICARE plans to give you a better sense of eligibility and how the plans operate. Costs are explained in Chapter 6.

TRICARE Prime

Overview

TRICARE Prime is a **fee-based, managed-care plan**. You will be assigned to a PCM who you will see first for any health needs (other than for urgent or emergency care). The PCM will either treat you or make a referral to see a specialist. Getting the referral set up normally takes a few days. Your care will be either at an MTF or a network provider, which means you will never have to submit a claim. Retiree families might have a small copayment for each visit; active duty families will not.

TRICARE Prime offers what is known as a Point of Service (POS) option. This allows beneficiaries to receive care from a TRICARE-authorized provider other than their PCM <u>without</u> a referral. However, this can be **quite costly** and should generally be avoided. **See the section below on the POS Option.**

Who is Eligible for Prime?

- Active duty service members and their families
- Retired service members and their families (stateside only)
- Activated Guard/Reserve members and their families
- Non-activated Guard/Reserve members and their families who qualify for care under the Transitional Assistance Management Program (TAMP)
- Retired Guard/Reserve members after age 60 and their families
- Survivors of deceased sponsors
- Medal of Honor recipients and their families
- Qualified former spouses

Limitations

- Must live within a Prime Service Area (near an MTF) or sign a waiver for distance restrictions.

- Available overseas only to ADSM, ADFM, activated Guard/Reserve members and their families. All others can participate stateside only.
- Those over 65 must join TRICARE for Life (TFL).
- Adult children until age 21, or to 23 with qualifying college enrollment. See below for more on TYA.

Point of Service (POS) Option

The POS option allows beneficiaries of TRICARE Prime who are <u>not</u> active duty to see a TRICARE-authorized provider other than their PCM without a referral. This can be quite expensive, however, so use it judiciously. For a full explanation, go to: **tricare.mil/Costs/POS**

- There is a special POS deductible of $300 per individual, or $600 per family. You must pay this amount <u>before</u> TRICARE cost-sharing begins.
- Cost-share is 50 percent of TRICARE allowable charges, and possibly more for non-network providers.
- ***Warning!* POS expenses do <u>not</u> count towards your family's catastrophic cap, so there is <u>NO</u> <u>upper limit on your out-of-pocket costs</u>.**

Real Life Story: Childbirth Referral under Prime

In our Facebook group, one young mother shared how she scheduled childbirth at a network provider without a referral from her PCM. She erroneously thought her referral for prenatal care was good enough. This put her childbirth care into the Point of Service option, and TRICARE assessed her half the cost, about $13,000. Had she gotten the correct referral, her cost would have been $0. As of this writing, she is still fighting the decision, and we don't know the final outcome. It's been an uphill battle and would never have been an issue if she had gotten the proper referrals.

TRICARE Prime Remote (Stateside)

Overview

TRICARE Prime Remote is a **fee-based, managed-care plan**. It is intended for active duty members and their families when assigned to a remote location, far from any MTF. Members in Prime Remote will choose a PCM from within the civilian community. The PCM should be a network provider, if available; otherwise, you will choose a non-network physician. The PCM is your first stop for any non-emergency care. They can refer you for specialty care, if needed.

Like Prime, Prime Remote offers the Point of Service (POS) option. This allows ADFMs to receive care from a TRICARE-authorized provider other than their PCM without a referral, but costs will be much higher. See the section above for details on the POS option.

Who is Eligible?

- ADSM <u>must</u> enroll in Prime Remote if TRICARE Prime is not available where they live.
- ADFM, if they are command-sponsored and collocated with their sponsor.
- Activated National Guard and Reserve members ordered to active duty service for more than 31 days in a row.
- Activated Guard/Reserve family members if they live in a designated remote location when the sponsor is activated and continues to reside at that address.

Limitations

- Participant must live outside a Prime Service Area (PSA).
- Prime Remote is not available to retirees.

TRICARE Prime Remote (Overseas)

Overview

TRICARE Prime Remote Overseas is a **fee-based, managed-care plan** for active duty and <u>command-sponsored family members</u> in designated remote overseas locations. Because you will not be near an MTF, members will choose a PCM in the civilian community. Your PCM should be a network provider, if one is available, otherwise you will choose a non-network physician. The PCM is your first stop for any non-emergency care. They can refer you for specialty care, if needed.

Like Prime, Prime Remote Overseas offers the Point of Service (POS) option. This allows beneficiaries to receive care from a TRICARE-authorized provider other than their PCM without a referral, but costs will be much higher. See the section above for details on the POS option.

Who is Eligible?

- Active duty service members
- Activated National Guard/Reserve members
- Command-sponsored family members of eligible sponsors

Limitations

- Must live outside a Prime Service Area (PSA)
- Not available to retirees

TRICARE Select

Overview

TRICARE Select is a **fee-based, non-managed care plan** available worldwide to qualified members. You can see any authorized provider of your choosing without a referral. ADFMs worldwide can enroll in Select, if they choose. We have had reports in our Facebook group of ADFMs being pressured to sign up for Prime even though they prefer Select. If you are an active duty family member, you can enroll in Select, even if you are told otherwise. TRICARE Select offers greater freedom in choosing your healthcare providers, which is why some beneficiaries prefer it. If this is important to you, **insist they enroll you in Select** even if anyone is saying that you "must" be in Prime.

For retirees under age 65 living overseas or living in the States outside of a Prime Service Area, TRICARE Select will be the only enrollment option.

With Select, you will not be assigned a PCM, although you can choose to have a family doctor. You may see network or non-network providers. Network providers will charge only your deductible and cost-share and then bill TRICARE for the rest; you will not have to submit a claim. With a non-network provider, it is likely that you will have to pay the entire bill upfront and submit a claim for partial reimbursement. See Chapter 5 for our discussion of network providers, both overseas and in the U.S.

Who is Eligible for TRICARE Select?

- Active duty family members (ADFM)
- Retired service members and their families, under 65
- Family members of activated Guard/Reserve members
- Non-activated Guard/Reserve members and their families who qualify for the Transitional Assistance Management Program (TAMP)
- Retired Guard/Reserve members over age 60 and their families
- Survivors of deceased sponsors
- Medal of Honor recipients and their families
- Qualified former spouses

Limitations

- Active duty members, including activated Guard and Reserve, cannot enroll in Select.
- Participants over age 65 must join TRICARE for Life (TFL). Some exceptions apply. Read about TFL below.

U.S. Family Health Plan

Overview

USFHP is a form of TRICARE Prime: a **fee-based, managed care plan**. Like TRICARE Prime, enrollees are assigned a PCM who normally will be their first stop for care.

USFHP is offered through community-based, non-profits in specific regions of the United States. As of this writing, clusters can be found around New England/Eastern Great Lakes, the Houston-San Antonio area, the Pacific Northwest (including much of Idaho and California), the New Jersey/NYC region, and the National Capital Region. New locations continue to be added. You can find the current list of providers and regions at **www.tricare.mil/usfhp** or **www.usfhp.net**. Use the TRICARE Plan Finder tool to find out if USFHP is available where you live. Chapter 3 explains how to use this tool.

Some USFHP providers offer benefits beyond the normal TRICARE Prime offerings. This might include vision care, dental, or gym membership. Providers set their own policy in this regard, so check with them to see what is available near you. Other than that, **pricing of USFHP is identical to Prime.**

Who is Eligible for USFHP?

- Active duty family members (**NOT** the AD sponsor)
- Retired service members and their families under age 65
- Family members of activated Guard/Reserve members

- Non-activated Guard/Reserve members and their families who qualify for Transitional Assistance Management Program (TAMP)
- Retired Guard/Reserve members at age 60 and their families
- Survivors of deceased sponsors
- Medal of Honor recipients and their families
- Qualified former spouses

Limitations

- Active duty members may not participate
- Until October 1, 2012, USFHP was available to Medicare-eligible beneficiaries, age 65 years and older. USFHP is no longer accepting Medicare-eligible members, but existing enrollees can remain in the plan.
- New Medicare-eligible beneficiaries, age 65 and older, must enroll in TRICARE for Life.

TRICARE for Life/Medicare

TRICARE for Life (TFL) and Medicare begin at age 65 for most people. Your health benefits can be used worldwide, so whether you are in the States or abroad, you are covered.

Chapter 8 covers these benefits in full. While Medicare works only within the U.S. and territories, TFL is available worldwide. Read Chapter 8 carefully for full details. Also join our Facebook group for discussion about this or visit our YouTube channel for informative videos. These resources and more can be found at **www.theTRICAREguy.com**

TRICARE Retired Reserve

Overview

TRICARE Retired Reserve (TRR) is a **premium-based, non-managed care plan** available worldwide for retirement-eligible members of the Selected Reserve and their families prior to drawing retired pay at age 60.

TRR provides comprehensive health care from retirement from the reserves until age 60. When the sponsor turns 60, the sponsor and all family members will migrate to plans available to other retiree families.

Who is eligible for TRR?

- Retired Reserve members under age 60 who are qualified for non-regular retirement and are not eligible for the Federal Employees Health Benefits (FEHB) program.
- Family members of qualified Retired Reserve members.
- Surviving spouses who have not remarried and surviving children if the sponsor was covered by TRR at the time of death. Survivor eligibility remains until the date the deceased sponsor would have turned 60 years old.

Limitations

- When the sponsor reaches age 60 and becomes eligible for retired pay, all family members will transition to other plans – such as TRICARE Prime or Select – subject to qualification criteria of those other plans.

- Surviving family of deceased sponsors will not be eligible if their sponsor was not enrolled in TRR at their time of death.

TRICARE Reserve Select

Overview

TRICARE Reserve Select (TRS) is a **fee-based, non-managed care** plan available worldwide for qualified members of the Selected Reserve and their families.

Who is eligible?

- Members of the Selected Reserve not on active duty orders who are not covered under TAMP and are not eligible for FEHB.
- Family members of qualifying TRS members.
- Survivors of Retired Reserve members if the sponsor was covered by TRS at the time of death. Surviving spouses cannot be remarried.

Limitations

- Members of the Individual Ready Reserve, including Navy Reserve Voluntary Training Units, do not qualify for TRS.
- Surviving family members are not eligible if their sponsor was not enrolled in TRS at time of death.
- Surviving spouses are not eligible if they have remarried.

TRICARE Plus

Overview

TRICARE Plus is an **add-on to non-managed care plans**, offering limited coverage at participating military hospitals and clinics. There is no cost for TRICARE Plus because it provides care only at the Military Treatment Facility (MTF) for which you have been pre-approved. Each MTF decides whether TRICARE Plus will be offered, based on their patient capacity and other considerations.

TRICARE Plus has several significant drawbacks:

- Enrollment is only for the MTF in which you are accepted.
- It provides priority access only to the primary care clinic of your approved MTF. There is no priority access for specialty care.

- TRICARE Plus does not cover <u>any</u> care from civilian providers. Unless you have other health coverage, you will be responsible for the entire bill for care received off base.

For these reasons, **TRICARE Plus is not a suitable plan for full family protection.** It should be used only to augment other coverage that you may have, such as Select or TFL.

TRICARE Plus can be a useful addition to any non-managed care you might have. For instance, if you are in TRICARE Select or TRICARE for Life and also enroll in TRICARE Plus, then you could be seen on base for routine care at no charge and still have coverage for specialists off base through your other plan. This can work both overseas and in the United States, if your local MTF participates in TRICARE Plus.

Who is eligible for TRICARE Plus?
- Anyone who is TRICARE-eligible and NOT enrolled in a TRICARE Prime plan, U.S. Family Health Plan, or a Medicare Health Maintenance Organization (HMO).
- For a dependent parent or parent-in-law, TRICARE Plus is the <u>only</u> TRICARE plan in which they can enroll. See Chapter 2 for more information about dependent parents and their eligibility for TRICARE.

Limitations
- The decision to offer Plus at any specific MTF rests with local commanders. TRICARE and MHS are not involved in this decision.
- You must inquire at the desired facility to be accepted into Plus. It is not transferable to any other MTF.
- TRICARE Plus should be only an adjunct to supplement another plan, not in lieu of other coverage. It cannot be used off base and does not include priority access to specialty care within the MTF.

TRICARE Young Adult (Prime Option)

Overview

TRICARE Young Adult-Prime (TYA-P) is a **premium-based, managed-care plan** for adult children of sponsors who lose their "regular" coverage at age 21 or 23. TYA-P works the same as TRICARE Prime. Beneficiaries have a PCM who will refer a patient to specialists when needed. Qualifying members can remain on this plan until age 26.

Who is eligible?

- Children of active duty sponsors in all U.S. locations and overseas (if command-sponsored).
- Children of retired sponsors in Prime Service Areas in the United States.
- Eligibility begins at age 21, or age 23 if enrolled full time in an accredited institution of higher learning. Eligibility ends at age 26.

Limitations

- Dependent children remain on Prime or Select to age 21 (or to age 23 if enrolled full time at an accredited institution of higher learning, and the sponsor provides more than 50 percent of financial support).
- Enrollment is not automatic. There are specific steps to take to sign up. Enroll at least 30 days before expiration of other TRICARE plans to avoid a break in coverage.
- Cannot enroll if the young adult child is eligible for an employer-sponsored health plan based on their own employment, even if they decline the employer plan.
- Cannot be otherwise eligible for TRICARE coverage through any other means.
- Adult child must be unmarried.
- TYA enrollees are not eligible for FEDVIP vision and dental plans.

TRICARE Young Adult (Select Option)

Overview

TRICARE Young Adult-Select (TYA-S) is a **premium-based, non-managed care plan** for adult children of sponsors after eligibility for "regular" coverage ends at age 21 or age 23. TYA-S works the same as TRICARE Select.

- Visit any TRICARE authorized provider. (See Chapter 5 for a discussion of authorized providers.)
- If you see a network provider, you often will pay less out-of-pocket costs, and the provider will file claims for you.
- You do not need a referral for any type of care, but some services may require pre-authorization.

Who is eligible?

- Unmarried, adult children of eligible sponsors
- Eligibility begins at age 21, or age 23 if enrolled full time in an accredited college. Eligibility ends at age 26.

Limitations

- Dependent children remain on Prime or Select to age 21, or 23 if enrolled in a full course of study at an accredited institution of higher learning, and the sponsor provides more than 50 percent of financial support.
- Enrollment is not automatic. There are specific steps to take to sign up. Enroll at least 30 days <u>before</u> expiration of other TRICARE plans to avoid a break in coverage.
- Cannot enroll if eligible for an employer-sponsored health plan based on their own employment, even if they decline the employer plan.
- Cannot be otherwise eligible for TRICARE coverage through any other means.
- Adult child must be unmarried.

Direct Care Only

Direct Care Only (DCO) is <u>not</u> a TRICARE plan. **It is a status assigned to TRICARE-eligible beneficiaries who are not enrolled in a plan.** There are few who should intentionally be in a DCO status. You are placed there when you have not selected a plan or failed to make recurring payments for fees or premiums.

Those in a DCO status can receive care ONLY at an MTF, on a space-available basis. Since many MTFs will not serve retirees or ADFMs not assigned to that MTF, they may decline to see you. DCO also will NOT cover specialty care, nor any care received off base from civilian providers. In short, you might have NO treatment options with TRICARE if you are in a DCO status.

If you have not used TRICARE for many years and are not sure which plan you are in, it is possible that you are in a DCO status without knowing it. In our social media groups, we have learned of three situations in which this has happened to TRICARE members:

- Beneficiaries who were enrolled in TRICARE Standard in 2018 when that plan was discontinued and who failed to enroll in a new plan.

- Retirees in TRICARE Select in 2021 when a new fee was implemented. Those who did not sign up to pay the new fee were removed from Select after a grace period and placed into a DCO status.

- Those in TRICARE Select who had been paying the monthly fee and reached their catastrophic cap. Billing of the fee stops when the annual cap is reached and might not have resumed the following year. Members in this situation find themselves unenrolled from Select if billing did not restart, even though they previously had been paying the fee.

- As this book is written in early 2025, we are still experiencing significant disruption in the West region due to the change in contractors. Members are being billed inconsistently, and sometimes the "automatic" monthly payments stop without warning. Many have caught this and called to resume payments; we are more concerned with those who did NOT catch it and unwittingly are falling behind on payments. They risk falling into a DCO status with their entire family.

If you are in this situation, **contact your regional contractor <u>immediately</u> to discuss your options.** At the very least, you will be able to sign up for a plan during the annual enrollment window in November/December. Your regional contractor can advise you if there are other opportunities to sign up. See the section in Chapter 3 on "Open Season and QLEs" for details about signing up for a new plan.

Continued Health Care Benefit Program

Overview

CHCBP is a **premium-based, non-managed care** plan that:

- Provides temporary coverage for those who lose TRICARE eligibility.
- Acts as a bridge between military health benefits and any new civilian health plan.
- Provides the same coverage as TRICARE Select.
- Offers temporary essential coverage required by the Affordable Care Act (ACA).

Qualifying members can purchase CHCBP within 60 days of the loss of TRICARE eligibility. Learn more about this at **tricare.mil/Plans/SpecialPrograms/CHCBP**

Who is eligible?

Certain beneficiaries can enroll in CHCBP when they lose TRICARE eligibility. The following shows the categories of eligible members and their length of coverage under CHCBP:

- **ADSM, released from active duty:** Up to 18 months
- **Full-time National Guard, separating from full-time status:** Up to 18 months
- **Member who is losing TAMP coverage:** Up to 18 months (See the following section regarding TAMP.)
- **Selected Reserve member losing TRS coverage:** Up to 18 months
- **Retired Reserve member losing TRR coverage before age 60**: Up to 18 months
- **Dependent child or spouse losing TRICARE coverage:** Up to 36 months
- **Former spouse who has not remarried losing TRICARE coverage:** Up to 36 months

CHCBP Limitations

- **If CHCBP coverage is due to separation from the military,** the characterization of the separation must be "honorable" or "general." Any separation that is adverse in nature would disqualify family members from CHCBP.
- **Qualified beneficiaries must sign up within 60 days of losing previous TRICARE eligibility.**

Transitional Assistance Management Program

The Transitional Assistance Management Program (TAMP) is not a TRICARE plan, but rather an assistance program for some beneficiaries when the sponsor leaves military service. For those eligible, it provides 180 days of premium-free transitional health care benefits after regular TRICARE benefits end.

Who is eligible?

Sponsors and eligible family members may be covered by TAMP if the sponsor is:

- Involuntarily separating from active duty under honorable conditions including:
  - Members who receive a voluntary separation incentive (VSI).
  - Members who receive voluntary separation pay and are not entitled to retired pay or retainer pay upon separation.
- National Guard or Reserve members separating from a period of more than 30 consecutive days of active duty in a preplanned mission or in support of a contingency operation.
- Separating from active duty following involuntary retention (stop-loss) in support of a contingency operation.
- Separating from active duty following a voluntary agreement to stay on active duty for less than one year in support of a contingency operation.
- Receiving a sole survivorship discharge.
- Separating from regular active duty and agreeing to become a member of the Selected Reserve of a Reserve Component. **To qualify, the service member must become a Selected Reservist the day immediately following release** from regular active duty service.

For those who qualify, the 180-day TAMP period begins upon the sponsor's separation. During this interval, sponsors and family members are eligible to use one of the following health plan options in addition to military hospitals and clinics:

- TRICARE Prime or Prime Overseas (where available).
- TRICARE Select (U.S. and internationally).

- U.S. Family Health Plan (in designated locations).

Other active duty programs such as the Extended Care Health Option (ECHO) remain available during the TAMP period. (See Chapter 4, "Special Needs/ECHO Program.")

Special Programs

There are a number of programs that are limited by geographic location, duration, scope of care, or eligibility. Some are pilot or demonstration projects to test potential future TRICARE benefits while others address specialized needs. Visit **tricare.mil/Plans/SpecialPrograms** to learn more about each one. These programs may be withdrawn, but others are often added, so the following list may be out of date. As of April 2025, the special programs are:

- Autism Care Demonstration
- Cancer Clinical Trials
- Childbirth and Breastfeeding Support Demonstration
- Chiropractic Health Care Program
- Combat-Related Special Compensation Travel Benefit
- Computer/Electronic Accommodations Program
- Continued Health Care Benefit Program (CHCBP)
- Extended Care Health Option (ECHO)
- Women, Infants and Children (WIC) Overseas Program

Additionally, TRICARE offers provisional coverage for various types of specialized treatment. This list changes frequently and has included such things as 3D mammography, platelet rich plasma, and ablative fractional laser treatment. For a list of current provisional coverage treatment, visit **tricare.mil/Plans/SpecialPrograms/ProvisionalCoverage** or call your regional contractor.

8
Medicare and TRICARE for Life

Transitioning into Medicare and TRICARE for Life (TFL) is a big milestone for many of us, but it also can be a time of great stress and confusion. How and when do you enroll? Do you need a new ID card? What is Medicare Advantage, and should you get it? Which doctors can you see after changing plans? These are just some of the questions that many people struggle with.

To those who are concerned, we simply say: Relax. The key takeaway from this chapter is this: *when you are enrolled in Medicare and TRICARE for Life, you have one of the best possible health plans worldwide!* You have access to excellent health care at generally no cost in the States and at a very reasonable cost throughout the rest of the world.

Medicare is first payer for most care within the United States. If there are any copayments, these are covered by TFL, leaving you with zero cost out-of-pocket – and you don't even have to file any claims! Overseas, TFL steps up as first payer. You will have copayments, but these are capped annually. The U.S. territories, which are in the TRICARE Overseas region, are considered within the United States for the purpose of Medicare, so you can use both Medicare and TFL within the U.S. territories.

The author himself transitioned into Medicare and TFL as this book was being written. We have led countless discussions about this process in our Facebook group. With these lessons fresh in our minds, we will walk you through the transition and explain how to use your benefits with this health plan.

Eligibility & Enrollment

Individuals become eligible for Medicare in one of three ways:

- Upon reaching 65 years old, for American citizens and lawful residents.
- After receiving Social Security Disability Insurance (SSDI) for 24 months, discussed below.
- Due to certain qualifying health conditions such as End-Stage Renal Disease (ESRD).

As you can see, it is possible to become eligible for Medicare prior to age 65, meaning that certain individuals can be on TRICARE for Life before age 65. A great reference for Medicare eligibility can be found at **www.cms.gov/medicare/enrollment-renewal/health-plans/original-part-a-b**

It is virtually certain that military retirees and their spouses will qualify for Medicare at 65 as long as the spouse is a U.S. citizen or holds a valid green card and has lived at least five years in the United States. **For foreign spouses** who do not qualify for free Medicare Part A, special rules allow them to remain in TRICARE past 65 even without Medicare. See the section in this chapter on "Non-U.S. Spouses" for further information.

There is a seven-month window in which to apply when first eligible, including the month that you turn 65 plus the three months before and three months <u>after</u> your birth month. **There is a penalty if you miss enrolling** during your initial eligibility; see the next section for details. TRICARE asserts that enrollment in TFL is automatic once you enroll in Medicare Part B, and it often is – but we <u>strongly</u> advise you to double check.

We have created a video about enrolling in Medicare & TFL. You can find this and many other videos on our YouTube channel at **www.youtube.com/@thetricareguy**

Age-related Medicare enrollment breaks down into three cases:

- **If you live in the States and are receiving Social Security benefits** (either retirement or disability), then you will be enrolled automatically in Medicare Parts A and B at 65. About two months before your 65th birthday, you will start receiving information in the mail about enrollment, plus your Medicare card. Read these mailed notices carefully – *and hold onto that card!*

  o If you do nothing at all, you will be enrolled in Medicare starting on the first day of the month in which you turn 65. Payments will automatically be withheld from your Social Security monthly benefit.

  o If you prefer to enroll in Medicare Advantage or don't want coverage at all, you will have to take specific steps. Follow the instructions in the mailers. (Advantage is discussed later in this chapter.)

- **If you live in the States and are NOT receiving Social Security benefits,** you will have to manually enroll because you don't have benefits from which to withhold payments. Sign up by visiting your local Social Security office or online at **www.ssa.gov.** You will have to make monthly payments until your SS benefits begin.

- **If you live overseas,** contact the nearest Social Security office, embassy, or consulate to enroll over the phone or in person. If you are already drawing benefits, your Medicare Part B fees will be withheld from that. If not, you must make other payment arrangements. More information can be found at **www.ssa.gov/foreign**

TRICARE beneficiaries who have been receiving Social Security Disability Insurance (SSDI) or railroad disability benefits for 24 months will automatically be enrolled in Medicare Parts A and B at the start of the 25th month. **Do <u>NOT</u> decline Part B** or you will lose <u>both</u> your TRICARE and Medicare coverage! This is true even if you live overseas. Once you begin Parts A and B coverage, you will be enrolled in TRICARE for Life (TFL). You will make monthly payments for Medicare Part B but will have no TRICARE enrollment fees.

Those <u>under</u> age 65 who are entitled to Medicare Part A and have Medicare Part B can choose to remain in TRICARE Prime or the U.S. Family Health Plan rather than Medicare/TFL, if desired. You will continue to pay the monthly Part B fee, but TRICARE will waive your individual Prime enrollment fee.

- Whether you keep TRICARE Prime or use TFL, your claims won't process through the regional contractor. Tell your providers to file claims with Medicare.
- Medicare will process their portion and then forward the remainder to TRICARE for payment.
- TRICARE will cover the remaining portion, leaving the patient with zero costs to cover.

Penalties

There is a penalty for delaying enrollment in Medicare Part B beyond the initial seven-month enrollment window. There are also some exceptions to this rule, explained in the next section.

- **By <u>not</u> enrolling in Medicare Part B at 65**, you not only forfeit Medicare, but **you also will lose TRICARE coverage**. You MIGHT be able to get limited care at an MTF, but this is uncertain. Many MTFs no longer serve retirees, especially those over 65. MTFs can no longer be considered a reliable back-up plan for retiree health care.
- If you change your mind and decide to enroll later, you will have to wait for the next General Enrollment Period (GEP). GEP is for those who did not enroll in Part B at their earliest opportunity. As of this writing, GEP is January – March of each year, and coverage begins the first day of the month following your sign-up.

- Finally – and perhaps most importantly – if you sign up late for Medicare, you will incur a **lifelong penalty** of higher monthly fees. The penalty increases the longer you delay. At this time, the penalty is a 10 percent higher premium for <u>each</u> <u>year</u> that you were not enrolled. For instance, if you sign up for Medicare Part B four years late, your monthly fee will be 40 percent higher than it otherwise would have been – *for the rest of your life!*

Many military retirees living overseas question why they should pay for Part B when they cannot use Medicare outside the United States. They might be in relatively good health or have access to affordable medical care in their foreign setting. We believe this is a shortsighted view. As people age, their healthcare needs increase, and affordable alternatives eventually will no longer be available. In many countries, expats cannot purchase foreign health insurance after a certain age. By then, you might find that the late-enrollment penalty puts Medicare/TFL out of reach. Remember, even though you cannot use Medicare overseas, your Part B enrollment gives you access to TRICARE worldwide with a low annual cap on your expenses. Furthermore, anytime you return to the States, Medicare + TFL gives you access to full healthcare at no additional cost.

For these reasons, our emphatic advice is to sign up for Part B at your earliest opportunity and remain enrolled for the rest of your life. The stakes are too high to exclude yourself from this valuable benefit as you age.

There is another quirk in public law that basically says that you cannot drop Part A if you are receiving it premium-free. If you do, you not only lose your Medicare and TRICARE coverage, you also will be forced to <u>repay</u> any Social Security retirement benefits that you have received to date! If you ever feel the itch to cancel Part A, research this carefully, and talk to SSA. There should be no need ever to cancel Part A coverage. It doesn't save you any money, and canceling can put you at risk.

Exceptions

There are certain instances that allow you to delay enrollment after age 65 without penalty. The first is for any Active Duty Service Member (ADSM) or Active Duty Family Member (ADFM) over 65. As long as the sponsor remains on active duty, they and their spouse can continue in their regular TRICARE plan and do not have to enroll in Medicare. As soon as military service ends, it is important to contact SSA and enroll in Medicare without delay to avoid a future penalty.

The second exception is when you or your spouse is working past 65 and receives coverage under a qualifying employer group health plan with 20 employees or more. Once employment ends, there will be a Special Enrollment Period (SEP) during which you must enroll expeditiously into Medicare. *Be careful with this provision!* Within our group, some members were advised by their employer that the company health plan was "qualifying," so they did not sign up for Medicare while working. They later learned that the employer plan was **not** qualified, and they got hit with a lifelong penalty for signing up late for Medicare. Do NOT rely on your company for this determination. Check with SSA to make sure your employer health plan qualifies; there are certain technical requirements that the plan must meet.

We can think of only one instance where it might make sense for an eligible TRICARE beneficiary to NOT remain enrolled after 65. This is the case of a surviving foreign spouse of a deceased retiree, living overseas. If the surviving spouse has lifetime coverage through their national health care system and does not expect to return to the United States, then there might be little benefit to remaining on TRICARE. They need to do the math and compare the logistics of coordinating their national health plan with TRICARE for Life (which remains in second-payer position). Making the two plans "play together nicely" can be challenging, while providing little benefit.

Non-U.S. Spouses

After age 65, virtually the only path to remain in TRICARE is to enroll in Medicare Part B, pay the monthly fee, and transition into TRICARE for Life. This works for any U.S. beneficiary who is entitled to Medicare Part A at no cost. However, a foreign-born spouse who lives outside the United States with no SSN and no U.S. work record may not be entitled to premium-free Part A. For such a spouse, it can be problematic to obtain TRICARE after age 65 – but not impossible. TRICARE hosts a page explaining this at **www.tricare.mil/LifeEvents/Medicare/NoPartA.** If this link no longer works, then do an internet search for **"TRICARE beneficiaries who don't qualify for free Medicare Part A"** and you should find current guidance.

In brief, the steps are:

1. Apply for Medicare using the sponsor's SSN even if you believe you are ineligible. The goal is to get a rejection notice which will be used in the next steps.

2. If you are unexpectedly approved, congratulations! Start making payments for Medicare Part B, and you will be enrolled in TFL. Read this chapter in full for information on your plan, and Chapter 6 for cost.

3. More likely, however, you will receive a **Disapproved Claim Notice** in the mail. Take this notice to the nearest DEERS or military ID office to update your DEERS entry and get a new military retiree ID card.

4. Since you have been denied free Medicare Part A, you are ineligible to enroll in TRICARE for Life. Instead, you may continue enrollment in Prime (if you are in the USA) or Select (anywhere worldwide). You can keep your plan for the rest of your life by paying the normal monthly enrollment fee. Call your regional contractor to enroll in a plan. If the customer rep is unfamiliar with this unusual provision, hang up and call again to get another support agent.

5. Read this book in full to learn more about how to find providers, obtain care, and file claims when necessary. Having a U.S. bank account for direct deposit of reimbursements is useful but not required.

Procedures may vary if you are a divorced ex-spouse under the 20/20/20 rule, a surviving spouse with deceased sponsor, or currently married to a younger sponsor who is not yet on Social Security or Medicare. Contact the nearest DEERS office or your regional contractor for details.

Types of Medicare Providers

There are three types of Medicare providers within the United States and U.S. territories. Your cost under TFL, if any, may vary depending upon the type of provider you see.

- **Participating providers** accept Medicare's allowed amount as payment in full. These providers bill directly to Medicare, with TRICARE covering the copayment. You pay nothing and will not have to submit a claim.

- **Non-participating providers** may charge up to 15 percent above Medicare's allowed amount. TRICARE covers this additional fee, so TFL members should have no out-of-pocket costs. Providers may or may not submit claims on your behalf. This is a question that you should ask when choosing a provider.

- **Opt-Out providers** do not participate in Medicare and are not allowed to bill Medicare. Medicare will not cover any of the bill. TRICARE will pay its normal 20 percent, leaving you responsible for the remaining 80 percent. In regions where access to medical care is sparse, TFL may waive second-payer status and pay the claim as primary payer, thereby reducing your costs. You should confirm this in advance of receiving care from an opt-out provider. In this case, you would pay the bill in full and submit a claim to TRICARE for reimbursement.

As of this writing, approximately 90 percent of primary care doctors in the United States accept Medicare. In most stateside locations, it is not difficult to find providers who accept Medicare, but not all are taking new patients. If you enroll in Medicare Advantage, however, you will be limited only to doctors within that Advantage network, possibly making it more difficult to schedule an appointment. Read further in this chapter for information about Medicare Advantage and Medicare supplements, and whether these plans make sense for you.

Using Medicare and TFL Stateside

If you obtain care within the U.S. or its territories, Medicare will be the first payer. You can make an appointment with the provider of your choice other than opt-out providers.

If you have previously seen this provider before joining Medicare, be sure you tell them you have changed insurance, or they will send the bill to TRICARE, and it will be rejected. They'll need to make a copy of your Medicare card for their records.

After paying its share, Medicare automatically forwards the bill to TFL, which covers any remaining costs, such as copayments. You, the beneficiary, will not have to submit a claim and will have no costs for covered care. The system works quite well; we have members in our Facebook group who have never seen a bill or paid a dime for decades under TFL.

You eventually will receive two different Explanation of Benefits (EOB) statements for your medical care. First, Medicare will send an EOB showing what it covered. It will show an unpaid amount, which is the copayment. *This is not a bill; do not pay anyone!* Later, you will receive an EOB from TFL. It will show that the Medicare copayment is fully paid, and there are no further costs for you to cover. Don't panic when you get the Medicare EOB showing a copayment; the bill is still working its way through the TRICARE system for final payoff.

Using TFL Internationally

Medicare can't be used outside the USA or U.S. territories, so internationally, TRICARE becomes the first payer. Overseas, TFL works very much like TRICARE Select.

- You can see any medically licensed provider without a referral.
- You normally will pay the bill upfront and submit a claim to TRICARE Overseas.
- You will have a 25 percent cost-share, until you reach your annual cap. After reaching your cap, you will have no further copayments until January 1 of the next year.
- If you find a network provider overseas (yes, they exist!), you can end up with a much smaller cost-share.

There is a broad misperception that TFL enrollees living internationally are switched to TRICARE Select. *This is not true!* The two plans work similarly, but they are not identical. An important difference, as of this writing, is that the catastrophic cap for Medicare is less than the cap for retirees on Select, so your out-of-pocket expenses are capped at a lower level under TFL.

If you are one of those old-timers who grumbles about having to pay for Medicare overseas "where it cannot be used", **please re-read the earlier section on Penalties.** There is real harm in not signing up for Medicare Part B when you turn 65, giving you worldwide coverage with TRICARE for Life. I am sadly aware of older vets who made short-sighted decisions that affected their access to essential care later in life. They opt out, lose their TRICARE coverage, and later find it too expensive to buy back in. These stories never end well, often resulting in an elderly vet with no health care at all, and friends passing the hat when they end up hospitalized with a critical need. Don't be "that guy" – sign up for Part B at your earliest opportunity.

Medicare Advantage

When you come of age to enroll in Medicare, you will find yourself bombarded with glossy marketing materials to sign up. In reality, these brochures are NOT Medicare, but rather Medicare Advantage. The materials are quite slick – they do not point out the difference between Medicare and Medicare Advantage (misleadingly named Medicare Part C), nor do they tell you that you have the option of doing nothing at all, which would result in your being enrolled in Medicare.

Advantage plans are <u>replacements</u> for Medicare, offered by for-profit commercial insurers. When you sign up for Advantage, you are no longer in "regular" Medicare; you buying a replacement and will be able to see only the providers in their private network. In other words, your choice of providers will be far more limited than regular Medicare. Depending on where you live and your need for certain specialists, this might make it harder to get appointments when you need.

On the positive side, Advantage plans normally offer certain freebies. They might reimburse the cost of Part B enrollment. They might offer gym membership, rides to your doctor, or vision and dental care. These are valuable benefits which, after full consideration, you might find worthwhile.

When considering Medicare Advantage, research each plan carefully (there are many), read reviews, and focus on your specific location to ensure that you will have access to the care you need. Remember: "regular" Medicare/TFL is highly portable and can easily be used coast-to-coast and worldwide. Your Advantage plan might not be so flexible, you may have difficulty in getting referrals approved. In our Facebook group, we have members who use Advantage and those who do not. Most people seem pleased with their decision either way, so it comes down to individual choice – just go in with your eyes open.

One precaution, especially for those who are just turning 65. Marketers of Advantage plans prey upon the ignorance, fear, and confusion of new participants. They make it sound like you must urgently select a plan or all is lost! They fail to mention that if you select no plan at all, you will fall under plain ol' Medicare and TFL, which serves the majority of the senior population extremely well. Don't fall for their trick of making it seem like you must choose between the different Advantage plans. When turning 65, if you make no plan selection, you will be enrolled in regular Medicare and TRICARE for Life, a combination that is hard to beat and serves the community quite well.

Medicare Supplements

A Medicare supplement (also called Medigap) is different from Advantage. Supplements cover Medicare expenses such as copayments and deductibles. **But this is <u>exactly</u> what TRICARE for Life does!** TFL is like getting a Medicare supplement for <u>free</u>. Medicare pays first, and any remaining amounts are automatically forwarded to TFL for payment, leaving you with zero out-of-pocket costs. TFL *is* your Medicare supplement, and **there is no need to buy a separate policy**; it would just be a waste of money.

Medicare at Sea

A little known fact is that your combination of Medicare and TFL can be used on cruise ships. This is not to say it would entirely replace the benefits of travel insurance, but this can be very useful coverage. If the ship is in a U.S. port or within U.S. territorial waters, then Medicare is available and would be first payer. TFL would continue to act as a Medicare supplement.

If the ship is in international waters or a foreign port when you receive care, Medicare will not work but you will still have access to TRICARE for Life. TFL will cover 75 percent of allowable costs, assuming the ship's medical department is an authorized provider. If you have travel insurance, then your travel policy is first payer, and you would submit your claim to them first. See Chapter 1 for a more detailed discussion on the merits of travel insurance and Chapter 4 for information about using TRICARE at sea.

Updating Your Military ID Card

The rules for updating ID cards for the retiree sponsor are somewhat different than for the spouse. For the sponsor, ID cards normally expire the month before turning 65 to ensure that they get a new ID card at age 65. While there are supposed to be standard procedures governing the issuance of retiree ID cards, in actual practice it may vary from office to office.

Since the sponsor's ID expires before turning 65, they must get a new ID <u>before</u> the 65th birthday, otherwise it may be difficult to gain access to a military base to get the very card needed for access. Our best guidance is for the sponsor to **get a new card in <u>the 30-day window</u>** before turning 65. By then, SSA and DEERS should show that they are Medicare-eligible. The new card should say "INDEF," meaning it will never expire; check this before leaving the office.

This 30-day window, regrettably, does <u>not</u> apply to the spouse. The spouse can apply for an INDEF card only AFTER turning 65. If applied prior to the 65th birthday, the new card still will have an expiration date and would have to be renewed one more time to get the INDEF card.

Most DEERS offices work by appointment, and some fill up their calendars months in advance. Others book appointments only one month ahead. You need to investigate practices at your local office. Even if they take walk-ins, there is a great chance that you will be turned away if they are busy. Go early in the day to increase your chances of being seen.

A case in point is the DEERS office at JUSMAGTHAI in Bangkok, which I personally have used. Gaining access to the facility without a current ID card can be difficult, so you don't want to be in that position. The DEERS office is by appointment only, but their online calendar rarely shows any vacancies. It can be hard to get them on the phone. This is a huge problem for retirees with a newly-married spouse whom they are trying to enroll in DEERS. Until they can navigate this obstacle, their spouse cannot enroll in TRICARE at all. Due to manning issues at the DEERS office, they often are unable to serve the retiree community at all.

The situation is bad enough that some have resorted to flying to Singapore, Guam, or Japan to use DEERS services there. This may be an extreme case, but it is hardly isolated. Our main takeaways are:

- Find the nearest DEERS/ID office that will meet your needs.
- Figure out their reservation procedures and book an appointment as soon as possible, but no more than 30 days before turning 65 (for the sponsor) or right after turning 65 (for the spouse).
- Have a back-up plan in mind, in case you find it impossible to get the support you need.

There is an online option that may allow both the sponsor and spouse to renew their ID online, saving a trip to an office. This should work both overseas and stateside. Visit the ID Card Office Online at **idco.dmdc.osd.mil/idco** for renewal or to make an in-office appointment. Once you obtain an ID card with an INDEF expiration date, it is good for life. You should never have to undergo this ordeal again.

9
TRICARE in the Philippines

THE PHILIPPINES HAS ITS OWN SET OF RULES FOR TRICARE. While this chapter provides tips and procedures for using TRICARE in the Philippines, it is important to **read the entire book!** Other chapters contain crucial information about health care benefits, filing claims, cost, and much more that apply in the Philippines.

The following resources are available to help you understand TRICARE special rules in the Philippines:

- TRICARE Overseas has a web page dedicated to using TRICARE in the Philippines. To learn more, visit **www.tricare-overseas.com/beneficiaries/philippines**

- Join our popular Facebook group **"TRICARE in the Philippines"** to ask questions and learn from others. Visit **www.theTRICAREguy.com** to find a link or go to **www.facebook.com/groups/TricareInPhilippines**

- Manila has the world's only VA clinic outside the U.S., located near the embassy. This outpatient clinic supports veterans living in the Philippines with service-connected conditions. For details, visit **benefits.va.gov/manila**

- RAO volunteers in the Philippines can help you navigate your TRICARE and VA benefits. See "Resources and Contact Information" later in this chapter to find these dedicated individuals.

- There is a special repository of forms that can be used to access care in the Philippines. Browse this listing at **www.tricare-overseas.com/providers/resources/ provider-forms/philippine-preferred-provider-forms**

Certified and Preferred Providers

One thing that differentiates TRICARE in the Philippines from the rest of the world is the use of "**certified**" and "**preferred**" **providers.** These designations are not found outside the Philippines. "Preferred" is roughly equivalent to a TRICARE network provider. "Certified" equates to a non-network provider. You should visit only preferred or certified providers in the Philippines, except in a medical emergency.

- **Preferred Providers** will bill TRICARE directly for medical care. This means you will pay only your deductible and copayment and will not have to submit a claim. The vast majority of preferred providers are located around Metro Manila, Subic, and Clark/Angeles City. There are very few elsewhere in the country.

- **Certified Providers** normally will not file claims for you. You must pay the bill in full and then submit a claim for reimbursement. If you are facing expensive in-patient care, ask the hospital if they will consider filing directly with TRICARE, so you will not have to pay the entire bill upfront. It is entirely up to them if they will do this or not.

- **All other providers** in the Philippines are NOT approved for use except for emergency care. **In a medical emergency, seek the nearest emergency care without delay.** TRICARE will reimburse the expense.

TRICARE Philippine Provider Search Tool

There is an online tool for finding certified and preferred providers in the Philippines. Learn to use this tool so that you do not have to depend on others to tell you which providers to see. We have seen far too many people rely on word-of-mouth about who to see and then are unable to get reimbursed because they went to a non-authorized provider. Do your own research! The list of Philippine providers changes often.

You will find the search tool for the TRICARE Philippines site at **www.tricare-overseas.com/beneficiaries/philippines**. Always use this tool when seeking care in the Philippines. Just because a provider was on the list before doesn't mean they still are. Always double check!

Using the search tool is a bit of an art. If you are not careful, it will appear as though no providers are available near you, even when there are. Here are some tips for getting the best possible search results. **Read these tips carefully and follow them precisely**.

- **The Provider Search Tool does NOT work well on a smartphone.** This is because there is a pop-up window which is hard to see on a smartphone. Use the search tool **only** on a computer.

- **If searching outside of major urban areas, enter only the name of your province.** Leave all the other boxes blank, such as the name of the town, hospital, or medical specialty; otherwise, you may get no results at all.

- **If you are in the Clark/Subic/Metro Manila area**, you can enter the name of the town to narrow down your results.

- If you don't get satisfactory results in your province, try searching in neighboring provinces.

- When you click "Search", a pop-up window appears with an X in the top right corner. ***Do NOT click the "X"!* If you do, the window will close, and you will not get your search results.** Scroll to the bottom of the pop-up and click "Show My Results" to see your list of providers.

- For providers with multiple locations, be aware that not every location is certified or preferred. **Carefully check the address of any provider** to ensure that it is the one that you want. If you get care at an unauthorized location, your claim might be denied.

If you follow these steps, you should be able to find a provider near you. Join our "TRICARE in the Philippines" Facebook group for further advice and support.

In a situation where there are no certified or preferred providers within a reasonable drive – for instance, if you must rely on ferry service – call TRICARE Overseas for authorization to use a non-certified provider for routine care. **Ask them to send the authorization in <u>writing</u> via TRICARE's secure messaging portal.** If questions arise later, having this written authorization will be a tremendous help to you.

Professional Fees

Professional fees are an aspect of the Philippine health care system where doctors and other medical professionals bill separately for the cost of their services. **TRICARE <u>will</u> reimburse professional fees**, but it takes particular care and additional documentation.

To claim professional fees:

- Some of our group members have said that a **Current Professional Terminology (CPT) code is needed for any procedure performed**, but this appears to be inconsistently enforced. We recommend including CPT codes to avoid problems. You can look up codes at **www.aapc.com/codes/cpt-codes-range**
- Include an itemized list of professional fees, organized by date. This will include:
  - Date of service
  - Name and specialty of doctor (e.g., surgeon, OB-GYN, anesthesiologist, etc.)
  - Description of service provided
  - CPT code
  - Billed amount, in Philippine pesos

- **Your health care provider may prepare this list, or you can create it yourself.** If you prepare it yourself, it should be typed and printed from your computer, <u>not</u> handwritten.

- **For anesthesiologist fees,** include the name of the anesthetic used and dosage or quantity and for how long.

- **Each provider who charges a fee should give you a detailed receipt** that includes their name, address or phone number, field of specialty, medical license number, amount of fee, and a statement of your diagnosis or a diagnostic code. Submit these receipts with your claim.

- As with all other claims, **call the TRICARE Overseas Singapore office 24 hours <u>after</u> uploading your claim**. Ask them to review your claim, page by page. They will tell you right away if they see any problems. Chapter 13 has more information in the "Follow Up" section.

If your reimbursement for care in the Philippines is less than you expected, it may be because the professional fees were not reimbursed. *Don't give up!* Continue calling to determine the problem and resubmit your claim. You should eventually be reimbursed.

Expert Tip: If you are admitted as an inpatient at a preferred hospital, your cost-share is capped at $250 per day for hospital charges **plus** 20% of separately billed charges. If the professional fees are bundled into the hospital charges, however, they would fall within the $250 daily cap, and you may end up saving money. If professional fees are separate from the hospital bill, you will pay up to $250 per day **plus** a percentage of the professional fees. Ask if professional fees can be bundled into the hospital bill to reduce your cost-share.

Pay with Plastic

In the Philippines, the rejection rate of claims is quite high, and once rejected they are tough to fix. One reason for these rejections is the historically high rate of fraudulent claims in the Philippines, where providers or beneficiaries (or both) try to defraud the U.S. government. Cash payment is a red flag because it is relatively easy to obscure cash transactions. When paying with cash, you can expect that your claim will receive greater scrutiny and is perhaps more likely to be denied.

One way to avoid this problem is to pay with a credit or debit card. Many hospitals and clinics don't accept credit cards, so **shop around within your community <u>before</u> a medical emergency**. This way, you will know where to go in a crisis.

TRICARE claims under $1,000 do not require a receipt. Nevertheless, we recommend that you submit a receipt with <u>every</u> claim to avoid extra scrutiny. **Denied claims can take months to resolve,** so anything you can do to streamline the process is worth the effort.

If you pay with cash, TRICARE will want a more complete paper trail. Here are some suggestions:

- Get a money order for the exact amount. Submit a copy of the money order with your claim.

- Withdraw the required amount of cash from the bank just before paying your bill and submit the bank receipt with your claim.

- Pay the provider with a direct wire transfer, online payment service, or cash app. Include evidence of this with your claim.

This added paperwork reduces the level of concern during the review of your claim and should help to resolve it faster. For more information on acceptable documentation for your payment, go to **www.tricare.mil/proofofpayment**

To streamline future claims, research within your community to see if there are any providers who accept credit cards. Do this BEFORE a medical emergency so you will know where to go.

Reimbursement in the Philippines

We are aware of three ways to receive your TRICARE reimbursement. Use the method that works best for you.

- **Direct deposit to a U.S. bank.** If you have a checking or savings account in the States, you can arrange for direct deposit, which reimburses your money quickly. The bank MUST have a U.S. routing number, <u>not</u> a BIC (Bank Identifier Code) or SWIFT code (international routing code). See Appendix A ("Establishing Direct Deposit") on how to set this up for yourself and your family members.

- **Mailed check in U.S. dollars.** If you have not set up direct deposit, then TRICARE will mail you a check. You can deposit a U.S. dollar check in the Philippines if you have a dollar account in a Philippine bank. There usually is a fee for depositing a check written in dollars, and it will take several weeks for the check to clear before you can access your money. You also can deposit a check in dollars to your U.S. bank account using a banking app on your smart phone, if your bank has this capability.

- **Mailed check in Philippine pesos.** If you do not have a dollar account, TRICARE can mail you a check in pesos. Be sure to indicate payment in foreign currency in block 13 of the DD-2642 claim form. Some banks are reportedly unwilling to deposit checks from TRICARE, so make sure to check on this before requesting this form of payment. Naturally, there will be concerns about the reliability of the Philippine mail system, which is another reason why direct deposit is a more preferred solution.

Expert Tip: If you live in the States and are planning to move to the Philippines, **be sure to keep a U.S. bank account open** to receive direct deposits from TRICARE. Otherwise, you will have to depend on checks mailed to the Philippines, which might be lost or delayed. Due to banking laws, it is very difficult or impossible to open a U.S. bank account when you are physically outside the United States.

Veterans Service Organizations

There is a great deal of assistance available in the Philippines for retirees, their spouses, family members, and survivors. Knowledgeable volunteers can help with obtaining VA benefits, filling out TRICARE claims, Social Security issues, reporting the death of a veteran, and other matters related to military service.

Veterans Service Organizations (VSOs) such as Veterans of Foreign Wars (VFW), American Legion, and Disabled American Veterans (DAV) provide support to veteran families. Veterans should make sure that their spouse is aware of this support so that they can get help in managing benefits. The VA maintains a list of VSOs at **www.va.gov/VSO.**

There are three Retired Activities Offices (RAOs) in the Philippines, plus numerous RAO satellite offices. RAOs have official standing with the Department of Defense, ensuring that they are properly trained and managed. The main RAOs are in Manila, Subic, and Angeles City. Any of these can direct you to a satellite office in your town or province. Contact information for the three RAO main offices is in the "Resources" section later in this chapter.

Besides general assistance with VA and TRICARE benefits, RAOs offer another very important service: **access to a military mailbox to receive mail from the United States**. You can pick up your mail at an RAO or have it forwarded to your home by courier. There is an annual membership fee to have the RAO receive your mail, plus the cost of courier delivery to your home. The next section describes how you can use this service to receive TRICARE prescription refills by mail.

Prescriptions by Mail

One of the great things about the RAO military mail service is that TRICARE beneficiaries in the Philippines can use Express Script's home delivery service to receive prescription refills by mail. You can either pick it up at their mailroom (at the Clark, Subic, or Manila office) or arrange to have refills forwarded to your home for a fee. Express Scripts can offer a huge benefit in refill costs and convenience. The FPO is authorized to receive mail weighing up to 16 ounces, but this weight limitation is waived for prescription refills from Express Scripts and the VA.

The only problem is that **Express Scripts requires a prescription written by a U.S.-licensed doctor**. This can be hard to find in the Philippines, so you may need to establish an ongoing relationship with a doctor in the States. Ask if they will do remote consultation with you to renew your prescriptions via telehealth or get refills when you visit the States.

Resources & Contact Information

There are a great many resources to help with TRICARE and other military benefits. Join our Facebook group "TRICARE in the Philippines" to ask questions. We are committed to helping people understand their TRICARE benefits in all situations.

This is the contact info for the three RAOs:

RAO Manila: No website available.

P&R Mansion, 1515 Sto. Sepulcro St Cor Pres. Quirino Do Ave, Paco, Metro Manila, 1007

Email: manilarao2012@yahoo.com

Phone: 632-8255-2729

RAO Subic: www.raosubic.com

P.O. Box 075
Olongapo City, 2200
Philippines

PSC 517 Box 5000R
FPO AP 96517-1000

Email: dir@raosubic.com or staff1@raosubic.com

Phone: 011-63-47-222-2314 or 047-603-0775

RAO Angeles: 1925mcarthur.wixsite.com/raoangeles

Retiree Activities Office
PSC 517 Box 2000R
FPO AP 96517-0021

Email: rao_ac@yahoo.com

Phone: 0915-965-0847 or 0939-847-7526

Global24 can help you manage your use of TRICARE within the Philippines. There are a variety of ways to get in touch. Their contact info is:

Address: Global 24 Network Services
P.O. Box 13892 Emerald Avenue, Ortigas Center
Post Office, Pasig City 1605

Phone: 632-8687-8656
Phil Toll-free: 1-800-10-456-2324
From PLDT: 1-800-1441-0576
Email: Support@GLOBAL24NS.com
Regional Office (Singapore): 65-6339-2676

The Philippines toll-free line is available to callers with service provided by PLDT (Philippine Long-Distance Telephone). We recommend that you use a calling app such as Google Voice for international calls, which can be very expensive.

Tips & Tricks for TRICARE in the Philippines

Over the years, members of our Facebook group, "TRICARE in the Philippines", have shared tips on getting the most from TRICARE benefits in the Philippines. The following is a selection of some of the best tips shared in our group.

- **Renew your military ID card.** Hospitals in the Philippines may accept your current ID card as proof of TRICARE insurance, although they might have to call the support center for verification. If you cannot prove that you have TRICARE, you will end up paying the entire bill and must submit a claim for reimbursement.

  o **Your TRICARE coverage is still valid even with an expired ID**, but it can be hard to prove this in the Philippines. Keeping your card current can make things much easier.

  o **Obtain a new ID card at the DEERS office at JUSMAG** in Manila (by appointment only). The ID office is in the same building as the VA clinic, **but the VA does not issue military ID cards**.

  o **For help with getting an appointment with DEERS, contact one of the three RAOs.** They can assist in making the appointment and also with preparing the application form.

- **Register your spouse and children in DEERS** (the Defense Enrollment Eligibility Reporting System). It is essential that **all** family members are registered. Without that, they cannot enroll in TRICARE. Your local RAO can help, or you may need to visit the embassy. If enrolling newborns overseas, read our instructions in Chapter 2. Keep DEERS updated with your current mailing address, email address, and changes in your family (e.g., birth, death, marriage, adoptions, guardianship, divorce, etc.).

- On a related note, it is likely impossible for any family member to be added to DEERS after your death. Don't think, "There is always time later." None of us know how much time is allotted to us. Make sure that your spouse and other eligible family members are in DEERS <u>today</u>!

- **Sign up for PhilHealth.** PhilHealth is a national insurance plan in the Philippines. All Philippine citizens are eligible, as well as some retiree non-citizens. It is considered OHI (Other Health Insurance) by TRICARE. When you use this program, you must first settle your bill with PhilHealth and get their Explanation of Benefits (EOB). Include the EOB with your TRICARE claim, and list PhilHealth as OHI on the claim form. See Chapter 13 for more information about OHI on TRICARE claims.

- **Do <u>not</u> include your over-the-counter (OTC) medications on TRICARE claims.** TRICARE Overseas does not cover OTC medications. If you have even <u>one</u> OTC on your receipt, this can cause the <u>entire</u> claim to be rejected. If you are shopping for both OTC drugs and prescription drugs on the same trip, pay for them separately and get separate receipts.

- **Use the TRICARE Philippine Provider Search Tool!** Do <u>not</u> ask your friends which doctors are Certified or Preferred. We repeatedly hear stories about members who were referred by friends to providers who no longer qualify, causing their claims to be denied. Even RAOs and VSOs make this mistake! Read the section earlier in this chapter about using the search tool. You will save yourself a lot of time, effort, frustration, and money.

- **Have access to lots of cash!** Many hospitals in the Philippines **require payment in full at discharge, and some are cash-only. Others may require payment at <u>admission</u>. Hospitals have even been known to hold a patient "hostage"** until the bill is paid while continuing to run up steep daily fees. Without cash, this can be a very stressful and costly situation. Members of our group have had to put a lien on their cars or other assets to facilitate release of their loved one from a Philippine hospital. Have ready cash at hand for this!

- **Establish a relationship with the nearest certified or preferred hospital.** The admissions process for first-time patients in the Philippines can be lengthy and arduous. Before ANY medical care is provided (even ER), the hospital will want to collect personal details, verify your financial status, and confirm your insurance. If you are gravely injured or ill, this waste of time can be critical. To avoid delays in an emergency, visit the business office of your preferred or certified hospital BEFORE a crisis so that the enrollment/validation process is completed before an emergency arises.

- **In a genuine emergency, go to the nearest emergency room.** Do not waste time searching for a preferred or certified provider. Get your emergency care without delay. TRICARE will accept your claim.

- **Install and use a calling app.** Many of our group members avoid calling the TRICARE regional office due to the cost of international calls. With a VOIP phone app, calls to the TRICARE Singapore office cost about two cents per minute, and toll-free numbers to the U.S. may be free. Search in your app store for a calling app to save money. This can be installed on a smartphone or computer.

  Calling apps are useful for more than just calling TRICARE. You can use them to call Social Security, DEERS, Medicare, your U.S. bank, IRS, and more. Having this set up in advance can be a BIG savings and a lifesaver in some situations.

Final tip: Practice, practice, practice! Using your TRICARE benefits is a life-skill that can be learned. The best time to learn is during a non-critical situation. A small claim for routine care is the perfect opportunity to try out your benefits and submit a claim. You can familiarize yourself with the process and make a mistake or two until you get it right. You don't want to be doing this for the first time during a medical emergency for yourself or a loved one. Reading this book is a great start but, **until you try it for yourself. you truly will not understand the process.**

10
VA and TRICARE

IT IS NOT UNCOMMON FOR PEOPLE TO CONFUSE TRICARE with the health benefits offered under the Department of Veterans Affairs (VA). We see this frequently in news articles, online discussions, and even in correspondence with Congressional representatives who ought to know better. **VA and TRICARE are completely separate. Their health plans differ in terms of eligibility, authorizing legislation, medical services, access, portability, and cost.** Yet many military retirees are eligible for both TRICARE and VA health benefits and jump back and forth between the two to suit their needs.

To contrast VA eligibility with TRICARE:

- Veterans can get access to VA health care by means of a disability rating, also known as a service-connected disability (SCD).

- Even without an SCD, veterans can obtain VA health care based on their military service, financial/housing status, or other considerations.

- TRICARE is primarily for active duty, reservists, retirees, and their families. No disability rating is needed. Most non-retired vets are not eligible for TRICARE.

- CHAMPVA, a VA health program for family members of certain disabled veterans, cannot be used by anyone who is eligible for TRICARE. Most readers of this book are ineligible for CHAMPVA. One exception is that gray area retiree families are eligible, until the sponsor turns 60.

Applying for VA disability can be an arduous process that takes months or even years, often requiring evidence from one's medical history. However, one can apply for VA Health Care **in just minutes** without having to demonstrate an SCD. There is no review of your military medical record, no panel of doctors assessing your claim, no medical exam, and no drawn-out litigation. Acceptance into VA Health Care can expand one's health care options in addition to TRICARE.

VA Priority Groups

The VA Health Care program uses priority groups to allocate care to veterans. Your priority group determines what care you may be eligible for and your co-payment, if any. There are eight priority groups: Priority Group 1 gives the highest precedence for care and no copayments. Priority Groups 6-8 have lower precedence and charge copayments for most types of care. See **www.va.gov/health-care/eligibility/priority-groups** for more information.

Priority groups consider a number of factors, including:
- Your military service history
- Disability rating
- Your income, assets, housing, and family structure
- Whether or not you qualify for Medicaid
- Other benefits you may be receiving, such as VA pension

Veterans with low income or service-connected disabilities are assigned higher precedence (a lower-number group). Those with higher income and no SCD are assigned lesser precedence (a higher-number group). This determination will affect what care you can get through VA and at what cost.

VA Health Care

Medical benefits under VA Health Care may be 100% free or come with small copayments, depending on the priority group and other factors. VA Health Care can be used only within the United States and U.S. territories except for issues related to

SCDs. For treatment of SCDs and possible aggravating conditions, veterans can receive care overseas through the VA Foreign Medical Program (FMP), which is discussed later in this chapter. For details, visit **www.va.gov/health-care**

During the application process, the VA will conduct a **Geographic Means Test**. This assesses your financial means based on your ZIP Code, income, and number of dependents. You are eligible to enroll in VA Health Care if **all** of the following are true:

- You fall within the income limit for your location, **and**
- You served in the active military (including activation in the National Guard or Reserves by federal order), **and**
- You were not dishonorably discharged, **and**
- You meet **at least one** of these service requirements:
  - You served before September 7, 1980, **or**
  - You served at least 24 consecutive months or for your full active-duty period, **or**
  - You were discharged for a hardship (early out), **or**
  - You were discharged for an SCD.

Time spent on active duty for training does not count toward the service requirements.

To apply, fill out and submit VA Form 10-10EZ, which can be found at **www.va.gov/health-care/**. This simple form can be completed in minutes. If approved, you will get a phone call for program orientation, assigning you to a VA primary care doctor. Call 1-877-222-8387 to discuss your eligibility.

After your orientation call, you will meet with your VA doctor who will review your medical history, determine if any specialty appointments are needed, and enter your current prescriptions into the VA system. **Even with VA Health Care, you will retain all of your TRICARE benefits** and can use either one for any given claim. VA Health Care does not count as

Other Health Insurance (OHI) by TRICARE, meaning that TRICARE can continue to be first payer, if you so choose.

If you already receive disability care at the VA, enrollment in VA Health Care can provide you with an even wider range of healthcare choices. **See my real life story in Chapter 4 about obtaining hearing aids** through VA Health Care which saved me over $4,000.

Outside the USA and U.S. territories, there are two options for receiving care from the VA.

- There is a VA Outpatient Clinic near the U.S. embassy in Manila. This is intended mainly for veterans residing in the Philippines and may be impossible for others to use. Chapter 9 has further information on this clinic.
- VA has a program of international care known as the Foreign Medical Program (FMP). This is strictly limited to your rated SCDs and possibly conditions that aggravate an SCD. It is not the full-service health care that you might receive in the States. The next sections discuss FMP and how it interacts with TRICARE.

Foreign Medical Program

Under the VA **Foreign Medical Program (FMP),** disabled vets overseas can see civilian providers, pay out-of-pocket, and submit a claim for reimbursement. You may even find providers who will bill directly to VA, with no need for you to pay upfront. FMP covers only SCDs or certain aggravating conditions; it does not provide full health care. **You must pre-register to use FMP, so enroll before the need arises.** The approval process may take some time, so start early. Visit **www.va.gov/communitycare/programs/veterans/ fmp/index.asp** for further information.

Besides seeking care for SCDs, FMP may also cover care for conditions known to aggravate the SCD. For instance, if you are rated for PTSD but also have depression which worsens the PTSD, then FMP might cover treatment for depression even if it is not a rated condition. Finally, if you are receiving care as part of the Veteran Readiness and Employment (VR&E) program, this care also may be covered by FMP. Contact the VA to get a determination for your specific case. It is important that the determination letter spells out precisely the conditions for which you are authorized care, so this will be honored through FMP.

Using FMP with TRICARE

Valid claims under FMP will be fully reimbursed, but the process is slow, taking up to a year. TRICARE is faster but reimburses only around 75 percent after deductible and copayments. Over the years, different strategies have emerged to get the most bang for your buck.

1. File with FMP to get all your money back. For larger claims, this is challenging since you must cover the cost out-of-pocket for an extended period.

2. File with TRICARE to get money back faster. This works well, but vets chafe at leaving money on the table, since TRICARE has copayments, while FMP does not.

3. A blend of the two, which is to file with TRICARE first, get the bulk of your money reimbursed in a matter of weeks or months, and then file a second claim with FMP to get back the remainder.

Option 3 proved to be quite popular with disabled retirees but, regrettably, some abused the system by submitting claims for the full amount under both programs, getting refunded twice for the same care. This is, of course, illegal but was done frequently enough that the U.S. government was compelled to tighten up against this fraud.

In 2024, TRICARE changed the DD 2642 claim form to list FMP as "Other Health Insurance" (OHI). Even though FMP is not an insurance program – it is a veterans' benefit – calling it

145

OHI forces those in the FMP program to file <u>first</u> with FMP, even if they would prefer the faster solution of filing through TRICARE. This would appear to take away options 2 and 3 from the list above.

This interpretation of lumping FMP into the category of OHI does not sit well with the expat veteran community. It feels as though TRICARE is penalizing them for having a disability, removing the option to file with TRICARE first as any non-disabled vet is allowed to do. One solution that quickly emerged is simply to avoid enrollment in FMP. If you don't sign up, then you can truthfully say on the TRICARE claim form that you do not have OHI. But this comes at a financial cost, since FMP grants 100 percent reimbursement, while TRICARE does not.

Through calls to the TRICARE Overseas support desk, we get varied information. They have said on occasion that on the DD 2642 claim form, you should check the box for FMP OHI **if and only if** you plan to file part of the claim with FMP. If you check that box, then you will have to file with FMP first. If you do NOT intend to file with FMP, then do NOT check the OHI box; and then you can file with TRICARE as first payer.

In practice, however, this has backfired. Some vets who followed this strategy found that their claims were denied due to failure to report OHI. Don't forget: Even if you don't report OHI on the claim form, TRICARE has a long memory, and they know you have FMP from previous claims. Failing to check the OHI box results in denial of the claim whether or not you actually use FMP.

In short, there appears to be no good solution. The only path that seems to work is to file the claim with FMP and wait for up to a year to be reimbursed. The situation continues to evolve, so please join our Facebook group *"TRICARE Around the World"* for further discussion about this issue.

VA Dental

Veterans may qualify for VA dental care through their disability rating. On a very limited basis, dental care also may be available to the non-disabled community, such as for homeless vets. Many VA hospitals and clinics have a long waiting list for dental services. Investigate this locally if you are expecting VA to be the main provider for your dental needs. Retirees have the option of dental coverage through Benefeds/FEDVIP.

There is a program known as VA Dental Insurance Plan (VADIP) which is more widely available to veterans and their eligible family members. These are commercial plans offered at a discount through the VA to qualifying families. To learn more about dental coverage under VADIP and FEDVIP, please see the section on Dental Coverage in Chapter 4.

11
Prescription Refills While Traveling

AMONG THE MORE FREQUENT health concerns of military travelers is how to obtain prescription refills on the road. Travelers often wonder: *Will the medications I need be available on my trip? Will TRICARE pay? How do I buy them?*

The laws in each nation are different, and not all medications used in the U.S. are legal or even available in other countries. If a specific medication is critical to your health, you must carefully research the laws in your intended destination. Two questions are vital: *"Is it legal for import?"* and *"Can it be purchased in-country?"*

An important thing for retirees to bear in mind: When traveling, you and your family no longer have the SOFA (Status of Forces Agreement) protections that you once enjoyed as an active duty family. If you "slip up" and are caught with prohibited medications at the border, you are at the mercy of local authorities. Base legal is not going to intervene or bail you out. Take extra care to research local laws when you are carrying prescription drugs into another country.

ISOS – the TRICARE Overseas contractor – specializes in medical logistics worldwide. They may be able to advise you about your destination. The U.S. embassy in each nation also has a website with travel information of this type. Take the time to look it up.

There are many ways to ensure that you have the medications you need while away from home. Each of the following options is discussed later in this chapter:

- Bring enough medications to cover your entire trip
- Visit a military pharmacy
- Refill delivery by mail (Express Scripts)
- Retail pharmacy (TRICARE reimbursable)
- Retail pharmacy (non-reimbursable)
- Deployment Prescription Program
- Refill through the VA

Bring Enough for Your Trip

This may seem evident, but it bears mentioning: Bring enough medications to cover your trip. Don't assume that you can drop into any drugstore for a quick refill. If you will be on a longer trip and normally order a 30-day supply from your local pharmacy, ask your doctor or pharmacist for a travel refill. This can provide you up to a 90-day supply of essential medications.

If you have enough time before your trip, you can switch to Express Scripts home delivery which provides 90-day refills for most medications. It can take some time to make this transition, so don't attempt this change at the last minute. To learn more about home delivery, go to **militaryrx.express-scripts.com**

There may be limits on what you can bring in and/or how much, so carefully research each country that you plan to visit. Check immigration and customs websites and other official sources to learn the laws. Common things to watch for:

- **Prescriptions** must be in the original packaging including a label with your name, dosage, and quantity.

- **Over-the-counter medications** also should be in the original packaging that clearly lists the ingredients.

- **Quantity:** Some countries limit the quantity travelers can bring in. Supplies for over 30 or 90 days might be deemed excessive according to local laws. *Research this!*

Violation of import laws can result in fines, confiscation of the medication or imprisonment.

Some countries prohibit medications commonly used in America. In Japan, pseudoephedrine, which is common in cold and allergy medications in the United States, is prohibited. Codeine or tramadol can land you in jail in Greece or Saudi Arabia. Customs officers worldwide will be indifferent to your plight if you are found in possession of what they consider "contraband." Worse yet is when a traveler is given a chance to declare certain medications but fails to do so. The act of concealment can bring a harsher penalty than simple possession. "Know before you go" is the best advice. Do your homework!

Expert Tip: "Don't put all your eggs in one basket." Ask your provider to issue each prescription in <u>two</u> labeled containers, each properly labeled with your name. When traveling, split your medications between different bags, such as checked and hand-carried bags. If one bag is lost, you will still have enough on hand while you figure out what to do. Start your preparations well in advance so you can handle any unexpected challenges or delays.

Military Pharmacy

If, despite your best efforts, you need refills on the road, the cheapest way to obtain them is at a Military Treatment Facility (MTF). Medications obtained at an MTF are free, but there are some precautions to bear in mind:

- **Most nations of the world do not have American MTFs**. Even if they do, the drive might be too far to be worth it. Investigate this <u>before</u> your trip.

- **Many MTFs no longer serve retirees**. An MTF's priority is to serve military members and command-sponsored dependents. The decision of whether to serve others is made by local commanders at each base, not by TRICARE. Don't assume that they will help.

- **Some bases may have restricted access** at the main gate due to security concerns. Even if an MTF says that it will treat retirees, it may be impossible to get on base. Access can change on very short notice due to military operations, so always have a back-up plan in mind.

- Regardless of base access, you must **confirm whether the pharmacy carries your medication** and what sort of prescription they need from your doctor. Local practices may differ from what you are used to. Don't waste vacation time on a wild goose chase that might not pay off. Call ahead to find out.

As you can see, there are a lot of roadblocks and obstacles to this strategy. If you plan to refill a prescription at an MTF away from home, read on for a backup plan that likely will include the use of retail pharmacies.

Refills by Mail

Express Scripts, the TRICARE prescription contractor, offers mail delivery of refills. However, this is not a practical solution for travelers outside the U.S. who will not have a mailing address while traveling. Express Scripts will not mail to a foreign address.

For those living overseas, this can be a workable solution if you have an FPO or APO address, but each country differs in what they allow. **In Germany, mail delivery of medications is prohibited by law, even to an APO address.** Keep in mind that other countries may have similar laws.

If you will be visiting friends overseas, don't ask to use their FPO/APO address to receive your mail! In most nations, it is a violation of military regulations for a member to use their FPO/AFO for anyone who isn't part of their household. You would put your friend at risk of losing their mail privileges or worse. This is a matter that you must solve on your own.

Check the nearest Retired Activities Office (RAO).
Many overseas locations with a large population of military
retirees have an RAO at the U.S. embassy, consulate, or military
base. Depending on local policy, RAOs with an FPO/APO
address may legitimately allow use of their post office box to
receive medications on behalf of local retirees. Before traveling,
look for an RAO in your intended destination. In the Philippines,
use of the FPO address is widely available to retirees nationwide,
although this is intended mainly for residents of that country,
not for visitors. See Chapter 9 on how to use military mail to
receive prescription refills in the Philippines.

Retail Pharmacy (Reimbursable)

The most flexible option for obtaining refills is to visit a retail
pharmacy and purchase your medications locally. With a non-
network pharmacy, you will pay out of pocket and submit a claim
for reimbursement. Your cost may be less at a network
pharmacy, but they are hard to find or nonexistent in most
international destinations.

To file a TRICARE claim, you will need a receipt with specific
information printed on it. This includes the pharmacy name, the
address or phone number, date the prescription was filled, drug
name and dosage, quantity provided, and the amount paid. See
Chapter 13 for details on filing pharmacy claims.

Pharmacies in many countries will happily sell you any
number of medications without a written prescription. Use your
best judgement to ensure that you are getting the genuine article,
not a pirated or substandard product. "Let the buyer beware" is
our best advice. If you require a prescription from a local doctor,
TRICARE will cover the cost of this doctor visit.

The Ultimate Guide to TRICARE

Expert tip: There are smartphone apps that help find low-cost prescriptions but, as far as we know, these apps work only in the States. GoodRX and SingleCare are two examples, but there are others. If you are buying from a network provider, you cannot use both the app and TRICARE benefits on the same refill. Compare the cost of the refill in the app vs. your TRICARE copay and pick the cheapest option.

Out-of-Pocket Retail Purchase

On international travel, you may find that local pharmacies can provide your medications very inexpensively even without a prescription. This is not uncommon in less-developed parts of the world. When you do this, you are not likely to get the receipt that you would need to file a TRICARE claim, so you will end up paying the cost out-of-pocket.

With this strategy, simply pay for the medication with no intention of submitting a claim. This may well be your most affordable alternative.

Real Life Story: Retail Pharmacy Overseas

In Thailand, a 90-day supply of my cholesterol meds cost only $7 at my local drugstore, less than the TRICARE copayment I would have paid at a hospital. This was the cheapest option for me, even without filing a claim.

I was comfortable with this approach because I was able to build trusted relationships with my local doctor and pharmacist. They assured me that the brand I was buying was authentic. If you are in an unfamiliar setting, exercise caution with this method. The last thing you want is a fake medication that might do more harm than good. Make sure that you are buying from a reputable source and that the medications are genuine.

Deployment Prescription Program (DPP)

Express Scripts offers what is known as the Deployment Prescription Program (DPP). This program allows deploying service members and contractors/government employees with TRICARE coverage to bring as much as 180 days of medication with them. Provide them with your email address and your deployment mailing address, and they will contact you when refills are due to confirm your next shipment. Your doctor should write a prescription to cover your period of deployment.

It is important to keep your address and email current with DPP; they cannot send a refill until you have confirmed the order. They will email you a reminder. **Deliveries can take 4-5 weeks, depending on your location.** Delivery options are limited for medications requiring refrigeration.

DPP is not for vacationers or family members but is a great option for those traveling on military orders. Visit the Express Scripts website at **militaryrx.express-scripts.com**, click on "Benefits" and then select "Deployment Prescription Program" to learn more.

Refill through VA

Many veterans on TRICARE are also eligible for medical care from the VA, even without a service-connected disability. This can include prescriptions at little or no cost. Once your prescriptions are entered into the VA health system, you can obtain your refills by mail or in person at a VA hospital or clinic.

Those with service-connected disabilities may be able to refill prescriptions overseas through VA's Foreign Medical Program (FMP). FMP provides 100 percent reimbursement without the copayment that you would incur through TRICARE. This can save you a bundle on higher-priced prescriptions. Learn more about these VA programs in Chapter 10.

Real Life Story: Traveling with a CPAP

Travelers to Japan who wish to bring in more than 30 days' worth of medical supplies or medical equipment, such as syringes or a CPAP machine, must obtain a *Yakkan Shomei,* a type of import certificate. I was unaware of this some years ago and carried my CPAP in and out of Japan many times without the required documentation. This escaped the attention of customs, so I was never questioned about it. You should never depend on luck, however!

In 2021, I was traveling from Thailand to Seattle via Narita, Japan. I called ahead to Japan Airlines to ask if my CPAP was excluded from my limit of carry-on items as it is in America. After I asked this seemingly innocent question, the airline staff became deeply concerned. They called back several times and asked for photos of my CPAP along with the serial numbers and a picture of the display with the machine powered on. They asked me repeatedly if I would be using it in-flight, which I stated that I would not.

When my family and I checked in at the airport in Bangkok, JAL representatives met us at the counter, had me unpack the CPAP, double-checked the serial number, put a special tag on it, and finally allowed us to travel. For that trip, we were not even entering into Japan; it was just a layover for the next flight. We got the go-ahead, but it was a nerve-wracking experience until we got that final approval.

Please don't let my personal experience deter you from doing the right thing. Had I not declared this piece of equipment – and their team had discovered it in my luggage – it could have been a real problem. The moral of the story is this: Every country has its own perspective on medications and medical equipment. Take nothing for granted. Do your research, follow the laws of each country, and enjoy stress-free travel!

12

During Your Appointment

IT'S TIME TO GO TO THE DOCTOR! Perhaps you are on a family vacation in the States, or you got sick in a foreign country. Maybe this is the first time that you've ever used TRICARE. In this chapter, we will walk you through what to expect. Whatever the situation, it's probably very different from the days when you simply walked into a military hospital, saw your doctor, picked up your prescriptions, and walked out.

Where Should You Seek Care?

If this is a medical emergency, go to the nearest emergency room without delay. <u>No pre-authorization is needed</u>, and POS fees will not be charged. Even ambulance fees will be reimbursed if medically necessary. Whether the ER is network or non-network, give them your TRICARE information. Most U.S. emergency rooms will coordinate with TRICARE for direct payment, even if they are not a network provider.

Some decisions about your care arise even before you get to the hospital or clinic. In every case, there will be paperwork to collect during your visit. Let's look at some common scenarios.

If you are <u>active duty</u>:

- You should seek care at a military hospital or clinic, if reasonably possible.

- **For emergency care**, if no MTF is nearby, immediately go to the nearest civilian emergency room. No referral or authorization is needed. Notify your PCM as soon as practicable after receiving care.

- **For urgent care**, visit an MTF or call the MHS Nurse Advice Line. They will advise you on the preferred course of action.
- **Routine care** for active duty members should <u>always</u> be with your PCM or with a referral.

If you are in a managed-care plan like TRICARE Prime and you see your PCM first, <u>relax</u>. You will either get no bill at all, or you will be asked to pay a small copay for the office visit. Your PCM will provide any referrals you might need, and you will not have to file a claim. When you work within the system, the process is quite simple.

If you are in a managed-care plan and get routine care <u>without</u> first seeing your PCM, this might be very expensive. By not seeing your PCM first, you are using the Point of Service (POS) option. With POS, you will have a large deductible and 50 percent cost-share. Worse still, it does not count towards your family's catastrophic cap, so there's no upper limit on how much you might pay. **If you are unable to see your PCM for a referral,** at least call your regional contractor. They might be able to give pre-authorization or other advice to save you some money. It is definitely worth the effort.

If you are in a non-managed care plan like Select or TRICARE for Life (TFL), there is no PCM. <u>You</u> determine which doctor to see and make your own appointments. If you are in the United States with TFL, you should make an appointment with a Medicare provider. Medicare will be first payer, TRICARE will be second payer, and your cost should be zero. If you are overseas and do not have other insurance, TRICARE is first payer, and you will use TFL exactly like TRICARE Select.

If you have any questions about who to see, contact the Nurse Advice Line at **mhsnurseadviceline.com**, available

24/7/365. They can point you in the right direction and might be able to arrange an appointment for you. To learn more about this valuable resource, see "MHS Nurse Advice Line" in Chapter 14.

There are many places – particularly overseas – where non-network providers will be your <u>only</u> option. **When you use a non-network provider, be prepared to:**

- Pay the <u>entire</u> bill before checking out (see Payment Tips later in this chapter).
- Collect all required paperwork (see next section).
- Submit a claim (see Chapter 13).

What Paperwork to Collect for Your Claim

You need to know what paperwork to collect during your medical visit. This will expedite your claim and might save you a trip back to gather what you need. **Documents do NOT need to be in English.** International SOS, the TRICARE Overseas contractor, can translate although this might slow the processing of your claim by a few days. I have submitted receipts in Thai and Japanese with no discernable delay.

There are three items to collect during your visit to use later in your claim: (1) a medical certificate, (2) an itemized receipt, and (3) a cash register or credit card receipt.

The medical certificate (also called a "medical report" or "hospital report") provides a description in clinical terms of why you were seen, your diagnosis, the lab tests conducted, treatment provided, and prescribed medications. It also may include diagnosis codes for your condition and the circumstances of your care (e.g., injury, acute illness, follow-up appointment, preventive care, etc.). This document <u>must</u> include your name, the doctor's name and medical license number, plus the name, address, and phone number of the hospital or clinic. It is <u>not</u> a receipt and will have no cost information.

Request the medical report at check-in so it can be prepared during your consultation. If you mention it at check-out, your doctor will have moved on to the next patient, and you will have to wait until they have time to prepare it. You can save time by mentioning it up front. There might be a small fee for creating the medical report or certificate. Have them add the fee to the total bill; it is reimbursable in your claim.

The second item to collect is an itemized receipt. This lists, in some detail, lab tests that were conducted, the doctor and nurse fees, hospital fee (if any), and all medications and supplies provided, annotated with the cost of each item. The itemized receipt **must be pre-printed with the hospital or clinic's name and address or phone number**. They can write all the other information by hand, but computer-printed is always best. **The itemized receipt should have a "Paid" stamp on it or some other indication that you paid the bill.**

The third item is a cash register or credit card receipt. This is a non-itemized receipt showing the amount billed, amount paid, and zero balance remaining. Official guidance says that you do not need a receipt for claims under $1,000, but I always include a receipt with each claim, big or small. This is just one more thing you can do to ensure your claim is approved the first time around.

Manage Your Care

We will not repeat generic advice about asking questions or assessing risk for any medical procedures. As a consumer, you should be prepared to address issues of importance to your TRICARE coverage. There is no blanket checklist on this subject; it comes with experience and through participation in our online forum while learning from the experiences of other members.

Here are some examples from our Facebook groups of how members managed their care within TRICARE:

- One member was told by his regional contractor that TRICARE would not cover the cost of an EKG during his annual physical without a statement of medical necessity. I had the opposite experience: my EKG was accepted without question. The doctor can include a statement of medical necessity for your EKG.

- For inpatient care, TRICARE covers the cost of a semi-private room. If you upgrade the room, TRICARE will not cover the additional cost. In many Thai hospitals, there are no shared rooms; even the most basic rooms are private. To avoid confusion, I made sure the invoice listed "standard room" and my costs were covered.

Over time, you will learn which questions to ask that are unique to your situation. If you need professional advice, call the MHS Nurse Advice Line, your regional contractor, or the nearest TRICARE Support Center if you are overseas. Chapter 14 has more information about these resources.

Payment Tips

The following payment tips can save you money and make it easier to get your claim approved. These are things that you should consider before the day of your appointment.

In Chapter 9, we discussed the pitfalls of paying with cash. **Cash payments can be a red flag to TRICARE claim reviewers,** especially in locations with a history of fraud. In many places around the world, cash is the only accepted form of payment. Consider any of the steps below to give paper trail of your cash and avoid any difficulties:

- **Withdraw the cash needed from a bank or ATM** and include the bank/ATM receipt with your claim.

- **Get a cashier's check for the exact amount of your bill and submit a copy with your claim**.

- **If you have a bank account in-country, pay via direct bank transfer,** and print a receipt.

- **Use an international payment service** like Wise to directly pay the provider from your U.S. bank account.

TRICARE says that you do not need a receipt for bills under $1,000, but we include a receipt for EVERY claim regardless of cost. It's easy to do and avoids problems later. Learn more about proof of payment at **www.tricare.mil/proofofpayment**.

If you are paying internationally with a credit card, it is common for vendors to offer billing in U.S. dollars or local currency. **Always pay in <u>local</u> currency, <u>not</u> in U.S. dollars.** If the vendor processes in dollars, they'll give a poor exchange rate to boost their profit. If you bill in local currency, then your card issuer or bank will do the currency conversion, giving you a better rate. I have seen differences of up to $50 on charges of $600. That's an astonishing 8 percent premium just to have the vendor calculate the currency exchange!

Before going abroad, obtain a credit card that charges no international fee. Most credit and debit cards charge a fee for international transactions. If you shop around, you can find cards <u>without</u> an international fee. With a **rewards card,** you can get cash or points back. In fact, instead of paying extra fees, you could be earning cash back on all your medical expenses!

Some members in our Facebook group swear that they lose money every time TRICARE converts currency on a claim. Personally, I haven't noticed this. If you use a credit card that charges no international fee and you specify to charge in local currency, then you will find that the reimbursement of your claim covers the credit card bill, less any hold-back for your deductible and copayment.

Below is my financial strategy for paying overseas with a credit card:

- I file my claims immediately after each appointment, so reimbursement normally arrives before the credit card bill is due. This allows me to use the reimbursement to pay off the card without incurring any finance charge.

- I pay zero international fees by choosing the right credit card. Most cards add around three percent for purchases overseas; by shopping around, you can find a card with no such fees.

- My card gives at least 1% back on medical expenses. Some cards offer even more, but watch out for annual fees!

- I decline the vendor's offer to bill in U.S. dollars, saving up to 8% on the expense. This practice borders on a scam because it takes advantage of the unwitting consumer, and the costs are not disclosed. This conversion rate scheme is becoming more and more common worldwide, particularly in areas frequented by tourists.

Expert Tip: Many overseas ATMs do the same "currency exchange trick" described above. While dispensing cash in local foreign currency, they offer to calculate in U.S. dollars. They have a number of ways of disguising this with confusing terminology but often phrase it as: "Avoid surprises – see exactly how much will be drawn from your account." **JUST SAY NO!** This scam can cost you $50 on a $600 withdrawal – it adds up! Have the ATM calculate in local currency, and your bank will give you a fair exchange rate when billing to your card.

13
Prepare and Submit Your Claim

THROUGHOUT THIS BOOK, we have presented many valuable benefits of your TRICARE health plan. Despite this, many people feel compelled to purchase additional insurance. Others do not bother to file TRICARE claims at all, leaving significant money on the table. With little effort on your part, TRICARE will cover medical expenses for you and your family. This is the "how-to" chapter where you will learn to prepare and submit claims so that you can put that money back in your pocket.

A Vicious Cycle: Why People Don't File Claims

Our unique vantage point of the global TRICARE community in our Facebook group allows us to see trends and issues faced by beneficiaries worldwide. One of the most frustrating things that we hear regularly is the litany of excuses for not filing claims: *"It's too hard"* or *"It's only a few dollars"* or *"They'll probably just reject the claim anyway."*

We've seen this pessimistic view play out repeatedly, so let's expose the fallacy. Say, for example, that you have an annual deductible of $150. This means your TRICARE benefits don't kick in until <u>after</u> you have a total of $150 in medical expenses for the year. But just having the expense is not enough – you <u>must</u> file a claim, so that TRICARE knows you had that expense. In other words, **you must file that <u>first</u> claim knowing that you might get little or nothing back.** This is why so many people think: *"Why bother?"*

This flawed logic overlooks one important fact: **If you don't submit the claim, you will <u>never</u> fulfill your deductible,** and you can go the entire year without getting ANY medical expenses reimbursed. Eventually, you may blurt in frustration: *"It's too late now! I should have started sooner!"* You've got a shoebox full of crumpled receipts and are no closer to grasping how the system works than you were at the beginning of the year.

This is not hypothetical. Members in our group confess to this exact behavior for years on end, leaving <u>thousands</u> of dollars unclaimed. That's money they could be using for groceries, car payments, travel, rent, and more.

In a similar scenario, many beneficiaries simply don't understand deductibles. They file a claim and, to their great puzzlement, get nothing back. Lamenting that "TRICARE doesn't work," they give up without realizing that the first claim fulfilled their deductible and that the next one would result in cash reimbursement. This is why we emphasize basic vocabulary such as the cost definitions we provide in Chapter 6. When people don't grasp the meaning of terms like "deductible" and "catastrophic cap", they end up making expensive mistakes.

As for the argument *"It's too hard"* – that's only true if you haven't taken the time to learn how to file a claim or find authorized providers. It might seem confusing at first, but after you do it two or three times, you'll see that it's not so difficult, and you will understand the process better. The only hard part is educating yourself – ***and you have the guidebook in your hands!*** Yes, there is learning curve, just like any worthwhile skill – but with practice, all your excuses will vanish.

Your medical requirements may be minimal while you are relatively young and healthy, but the clock is ticking; we all age. One day, you might need bypass surgery. Your spouse will suddenly require chemotherapy. Your child will get hurt riding a bike. These things come without warning, which is why you should learn – *today* – how to use your TRICARE benefits. You don't want to be frantically trying to figure this out during a family crisis.

It's heartbreaking to see people struggle because they did not learn to use their TRICARE benefits when they had time. What if it's <u>you</u> in the ICU, rather than your spouse? Will your partner be able to figure this out on their own? You are doing your family a disservice by <u>not</u> building this skill under more relaxed circumstances and sharing what you learn with your spouse.

You have made it this far – <u>this</u> is the money chapter. No more *"It doesn't matter"* or *"It's not worth it."* Get past that. Follow our guidelines and file your first claim.

Who Do You File With?

A few simple rules determine where to file your claim:

- **If you are enrolled in TRICARE Overseas,** file your claim with TRICARE Overseas even if you receive care while visiting the States.

- **If you receive care internationally or in a U.S. territory,** file your claim with TRICARE Overseas, no matter where you live.

- **If you live in the United States or U.S. territories and receive care <u>inside</u> the United States or U.S. territories,** file the claim with your home region. For instance, if you live in the East region and receive care in the West region, file with TRICARE East.

- **If you are on Medicare/TFL and receive care <u>inside</u> the United States,** you normally will not need to file a claim. The provider should submit the claim to Medicare (the first payer) but tell them that you also have TFL (second payer).

- **If you are on TFL and obtain care <u>outside</u> the United States,** file your claim with TRICARE Overseas.

167

It is important to file with the right contractor. If you submit your claim to the wrong one, they won't forward it or tell you to refile with the right contractor. They will go into a full 60-day review and then reject your claim for cryptic reasons. You won't understand <u>why</u> the claim is denied, even though it looks like you did everything right. It can take several calls to straighten it out and start all over again – IF you ask the right questions. In this type of situation, people often give up in frustration, eat the cost, and tell everyone that TRICARE doesn't work – all because they don't understand what went wrong.

How do you avoid all this stress and angst? By submitting a claim that gets approved the first time through, without going into that cycle of rejection. The rest of this chapter – and our One-Stop Checklist in Appendix D – focuses on how this is done.

How to File: Fax, Mail, or Online

There are various ways to file your claim, depending on your contractor: fax, mail, or online. **When you are filing claims with TRICARE East or West**, plan on mailing it in since they do not offer an online option.

When filing a claim with TRICARE Overseas, you can mail the claim or file it online. We encourage you to file claims online at the TRICARE Overseas web portal for reasons that we will explain later.

No matter which method you choose, **you can receive your reimbursement by direct deposit** to your U.S. savings or checking account. Funds will arrive about three business days after approval of your claim. If you haven't arranged for direct deposit, they will mail you a check, which can take weeks to arrive...or possibly get lost in the mail. If you are planning to move overseas, make sure to keep your U.S. bank account open. It is extremely difficult – perhaps even impossible – to open U.S. bank accounts when outside the United States.

A variety of forms for filing claims and managing your care can be found at **tricare.mil/PatientResources/Forms**

When to File

There are time limits for filing TRICARE claims:

- **For care received <u>inside</u> the United States or U.S. territories,** you have 12 months to file a claim.

- **For care received <u>overseas</u>,** you have 36 months.

Chapter 1 has a discussion of Other Health Insurance (OHI). If you have OHI, you must file with that policy <u>first</u>. They will issue an Explanation of Benefits (EOB). If you have any unreimbursed expenses, attach the OHI EOB to your TRICARE claim and list your OHI in Block 11 of the claim form. The OHI claim will take a while to settle, so don't wait until the last minute. Delay in resolving OHI is not an excuse for missing your TRICARE filing deadline. **If your claim is returned for additional information, you MUST respond within 90 days** or by the original filing deadline – whichever is later – or the claim will be denied.

Some people prefer to save up their claims and submit them all at once. We recommend that you file claims as soon as possible after you receive care. The longer you wait, the harder it gets. Paperwork disappears, you forget important details about your care, or you get overwhelmed as multiple claims start to pile up.

With a laptop and a scanning app on your smartphone, you can even create and submit claims from your hotel room while traveling. In a truly paperless process, I routinely scan receipts and other documents with my phone, mark-up the PDFs on my computer, sign electronically, and upload everything through the contractor's portal. By the time I get home from traveling, my claims are done – all without a printer or scanner.

Assemble Your Documents

Now it's time to assemble your documents into a claim package, which will include some or all of the following:

- TRICARE claim form (DD-2642)
- Hospital or doctor's report (also called a "medical certificate")
- Itemized receipt, marked "Paid"
- Cash register receipt
- Bank/ATM cash receipt (if paying by cash). This is especially important in the Philippines.
- OHI Explanation of Benefits (EOB) if you have OHI
- In the Philippines, details of professional fees. (See Chapter 9 to learn more about this.)
- Any other documentation to substantiate your claim.

You may submit foreign-language documents without translation. The TRICARE Overseas contractor has robust translation capabilities. This may add a few days to processing.

Complete Your Documents

Turn to Appendix D for our one-of-a-kind "One-Stop Checklist" to prepare your claim. All of the tips come from official sources. If you follow our checklist carefully, you can expect your claim to sail through approval in just a few weeks.

We want to highlight the single most important step in this process: after uploading your claim to the TRICARE Overseas claims portal, wait 24 hours and then **call to do a review by phone.** There are specific questions to be asked during this call, which are listed in Appendix D. This phone call is all-important and staves off catastrophic errors that can derail your claim and cost you months of processing time. Do NOT skip this step!

Keep copies of everything! Documents can get lost enroute, even with online filing. Protect yourself by retaining copies of all documents, at least until your claim is settled.

Filing by Mail

If you are mailing your claim, be sure to use the correct address. Mailing addresses are subject to change, so always double-check.

TRICARE East
TRICARE East Region Claims
ATTN: New Claims
P.O. Box 7981
Madison, WI 53707-7981

TRICARE West
TRICARE West Region Claims
P.O. Box 202112
Florence, SC 29502-2112

TRICARE Overseas (Active Duty claims)
TRICARE Active Duty Claims
P.O. Box 7968
Madison, WI 53707-7968

TRICARE Overseas - Africa & Eurasia (non-AD)
TRICARE Overseas Program
P.O. Box 8976
Madison, WI 53708-8976

TRICARE Overseas – Asia-Pacific, Latin America, Canada (non-AD)
TRICARE Overseas Program
P.O. Box 7985
Madison, WI 53707-7985

TRICARE for Life (U.S. & Territories)
WPS TRICARE for Life
P.O. Box 7890
Madison, WI 53707-7890

TRICARE for Life (all overseas regions)
Use the overseas claims addresses above.

Pharmacy claims (U.S. & Territories only)
Express Scripts, Inc.
P.O. Box 52132
Phoenix, AZ 85072-2132

Continued Health Care Benefit Program
TRICARE East Region Claims
CHCBP Claims
P.O. Box 7981
Madison, WI 53707-7891

Claims for NOAA Members (all locations)
U.S. Department of Commerce
Office of the General Counsel
Office of the Assistant General Counsel for Finance and
    Litigation General
Litigation Division
1401 Constitution Ave NW Room 5890
Washington, DC 20230-0001

Filing by Fax

TRICARE Overseas and TRICARE Dental Program (TDP) are the only programs that promote filing claims by fax. However, it can take up to <u>two weeks</u> to import a faxed claim into the claims processing system, whereas submission via the TOP online portal puts your claim into the processing system within 24 hours. If speed of processing is important to you, you should learn to file via the TOP online portal.

The following fax numbers are available for submitting claims:
TRICARE Overseas fax: 1-608-301-2251
TRICARE Dental Program fax:
    U.S. & U.S. Territories: 717-635-4565
    International claims: 844-827-9926 or 717-635-4520

We recommend calling <u>before</u> you send a fax to ensure that you have the right number. Next, call <u>after</u> sending your claim to confirm that ALL the pages have been received and are legible and correct. See our "Follow Up" section below.

Filing Online

With TRICARE Overseas, you have the option of submitting your claim via their web portal. One of the greatest advantages to this is speed: your claim is imported into their processing system within one business day. This differs from fax or mail, where it can take weeks for your claim to be entered into the processing system.

It takes a bit of computer literacy to master the portal. At a minimum, you'll need to know how to scan, merge documents, and upload files via the contractor's website. If you don't have such skills, find someone who can teach you or assist with the process. See Chapter 14 for sources of local assistance.

Besides the benefit of faster reimbursement, another advantage of online filing is that you can find and fix problems early in the process. Read "Follow Up" below about how to conduct a telephone review of your claim and to <u>instantly</u> resolve any problems that are found BEFORE your claim enters the formal review process.

Follow Up: How to Avoid Claim Rejections

If I had to pick just <u>one thing</u> to make the TRICARE Overseas claim process go smoothly, it would be this: **After submitting your claim online, call them the next business day (after waiting a minimum of 24 hours).** A customer support representative will review your claim over the phone. If they find a problem, it can be fixed during the call or by sending more documentation via the portal. Earlier I wrote that I have never had a claim rejected. That does not mean I always get it perfect on the first try. What it means is that I call the next business day and immediately fix any problems they find. With this one step I generally get reimbursed within 21 days, but some take longer.

When you call, you need to ask:
1. **Did you receive my claim?**
2. **What pages do you see?** *(Compare this to your copies to confirm that everything is there.)*
3. **Are all pages legible?** *(Pages sometimes become garbled in online submissions.)*
4. **Do you see any problems?**
5. Lastly, **confirm that the payment will be sent to <u>you</u>,** not to the health care provider.

These steps can prevent your claim from going into a rejection cycle. It seems to take eight weeks or more to reject a claim, and then you receive a cryptic notice such as: "Requested information not provided." This does not mean that they asked for something that you failed to provide (since we have never seen them ask for anything during the claims process). It means that your initial submission was deficient for some reason, and it is up to you to figure out what went wrong.

I am a big fan of TRICARE and want everyone to have as positive an experience as I have had. The best thing to do is to not let a claim go into that rejection cycle in the first place. To achieve this, make that follow-up call and fix any problems at the very <u>start</u> of the process. Don't wait eight weeks or more for a rejection, only to have to start all over again. **Follow our One-Stop Checklist** in Appendix D, wait at least 24 hours, and then make that follow-up call. *You can do this!*

Fixing Problems with Your Claim

When you call after submitting your claim, what do you do if a problem is found? In most cases, you will <u>not</u> have to redo the entire claim; simply submit any additional documentation that is requested. This can be a very quick process via the contractor's portal, even if you did not originally submit your claim through the portal. Each contractor has a Messaging Center where you can submit documents. **When you call, be sure to get the claim number and include it in your message with the new documents.** This is absolutely essential.

With TRICARE Overseas, if you submit your claim via the online portal, you will find a confirmation message with your claim number in the Messaging Center. Click "reply" on the confirmation message, attach any new documents requested, and send. The documents will be added to your claim package.

As you did with the original claim package, wait 24 hours, and then call to make sure the additional documents were received, are legible, and have been added to your claim. If they see no further problems, you can be 99% sure that your claim will be quickly paid as long as it was for a covered condition.

Pharmacy Claims

Pharmacy claims are similar to other TRICARE claims. Use the same claim form, DD Form 2642, and check "Pharmacy" in Box 8b. There are specific requirements for a pharmacy receipt:

- **Items that must be typed or computer printed on the pharmacy receipt include the following:** pharmacy name, date the prescription was filled, drug name and dosage, quantity provided, and the amount paid by the beneficiary.

- **Items that can be handwritten on the receipt include:** the prescription number, pharmacy address, doctor's name, pharmacist's signature, retail price, and the amount paid by other health insurance (OHI).

There are different mailing addresses to send in pharmacy claims, depending on where the prescription was obtained. As always, double-check these addresses in case they might have changed. **In the United States or U.S. territories,** mail your pharmacy claim to Express Scripts at:

Express Scripts, Inc.
P.O. Box 52132
Phoenix AZ 85072-2132

For international pharmacy claims, use the applicable address for TRICARE Overseas claims in the "Filing By Mail" section earlier in this chapter.

Dental Claims

Forms and information about filing TRICARE dental claims can be found at **tricare.mil/FormsClaims/Claims/Dental**

For the Active Duty Dental Program, send the claim form and supporting documentation to:

United Concordia
Claims Processing
P.O. Box 69429
Harrisburg, PA 17106-9429

For the TRICARE Dental Program (U.S. & territories), mail or fax your claim to:

United Concordia
TRICARE Dental Program
P.O. Box 69451
Harrisburg, PA 17106
Fax: 717-635-4565

For the TRICARE Dental Program (International), mail or fax your claim form to:

United Concordia
TRICARE Dental Program
P.O. Box 69452
Harrisburg, PA 17106
Fax: 844-827-9926 (toll-free) or 717-635-4520

For FEDVIP dental plans, visit the website of your dental administrator for information on how to file claims.

Filing Complaints

Despite your best efforts, there is always a chance that something will go wrong. Perhaps a claim is denied or approved for a lesser amount than expected. Maybe you didn't receive the professional and courteous treatment that you deserve. What should you do next?

The first thing to do is **pick up the phone and call!** Nine times out of ten, your issue can be resolved over the phone. They will either figure out what went wrong and give you a chance to fix it, or they may clearly explain why your claim was denied, so you will understand that an appeal will not help. Several times, my reimbursement was less than expected. After discussing it by phone, they recognized their mistake and sent the remaining money. I didn't have to submit any paperwork.

If you are unable to resolve the matter by phone, you might be able to **find an advocate** who can help. Such advocates include:

- **Ombudsman or patient advocate** at hospitals, clinics, and other care centers. Their role is to help patients resolve issues within a facility when they arise.
- **Beneficiary Counseling and Assistance Coordinator (BCAC)** whose role is to help with questions about TRICARE eligibility, enrollment, referrals/authorizations, and claims.

Learn more about advocates and other sources of assistance in Chapter 14.

If after all of this, you are still at an impasse, then it's time to **submit a formal complaint**. In TRICARE, there are two kinds:

- **Appeal:** If you were denied care or payment to which you believe that you are entitled.

- **Grievance:** If you are not satisfied with the quality of care received, the behavior of any specific person in the TRICARE system, or any other non-appealable issue.

Appeals are broken down into four types:

- **Factual appeal** is when you are denied payment for services or supplies that you received.

- **Medical necessity appeal** is when you are denied authorization for care or services because TRICARE feels it isn't medically necessary.

- **Pharmacy appeal** is when you don't agree with a decision about your pharmacy benefit.

- **Medicare-TRICARE appeal** applies if you're eligible for both TRICARE and Medicare, and Medicare denies your services or supplies. This would not apply to an overseas claim since Medicare cannot be used overseas.

Examples of grievances include:

- **The quality of care** given by a provider, such as inappropriate care, not enough care, or poor results.

- **The attitude or behavior** of providers and their staff.

- **Incorrect information** provided to you.

- **Delays or errors** in processing authorizations.

- **Patient safety issues** at a facility.

- **Privacy concerns.**

Submit grievances and appeals to the contractor who is handling your claim. Each regional contractor has its own forms and procedures for complaints. Search for "complaint" using the search function on your regional contractor's website. It will lead you to their guidance for submitting a complaint.

Expert tip: If you plan to call your regional contractor with a question, do <u>not</u> message them before calling. This could backfire. TRICARE Contractors are allowed a full 30 days to answer your written question. If you call during that 30-day period, they will say: *"You've already written to us about this. Give us 30 days to reply,"* and they will not answer your question over the phone. It's infuriating! I've learned to **call without messaging first**. Once I have an answer, I ask them to send a response through the Secure Messaging Center, so I have the answer in writing.

Third Party Liability

Under federal law, the government has the right to recover the cost of care if your injury was due to the intentional or accidental actions of another. Recovery of costs may be from the third party or from the beneficiary if the care has already been reimbursed by third-party insurance. This right of cost-recovery applies even if the care was provided at an MTF.

Chapter 10, Section 5 of the TRICARE Operations Manual 6010.56-M, "Claims Adjustments and Recoupments" says:

The Federal Medical Care Recovery Act (FMCRA) provides for the recovery of the costs of medical care furnished by the United States to a person suffering a disease or injury caused by the action or negligence of some third person. Under this act, the United States has a right to recover the reasonable value of the care and treatment from the person(s) responsible for the injury. For TRICARE beneficiaries, this includes care that may be received by the beneficiary at a Uniformed Services facility or under TRICARE, or both. The FMCRA applies only to illness or injury (including work-related injuries) caused by a third party, either intentionally or negligently, or injuries caused by a third party's failure to act when a duty to act could be implied.

If TRICARE suspects your condition involves third-party liability, they will send you DD Form 2527, "Statement of Personal Injury – Possible Third Party Liability Form." This can be triggered either by the nature of your injury or by the diagnostic codes used by your health care provider. In these cases, your Regional Contractor will send you DD Form 2527 to clarify the circumstances. *Do not ignore this form!* **Your claim will be placed on hold and <u>canceled</u>** within 35 days if you fail to respond.

Ask your provider to explain the ICD codes used for your diagnosis. Work with them to clarify that the injury was not due to an accident, and no third party was involved. If this can be done when care is provided, you may avoid this additional step and possible delay in the processing of your claim.

14
Additional Help & Contact Info

THERE ARE NUMEROUS RESOURCES to help you find the care that you need, navigate your benefits, and submit claims. Take advantage of the many free services that are offered. There is no need to figure everything out alone or reinvent the wheel.

The TRICARE Website

The official TRICARE website is **www.tricare.mil**. You do not need to log in or create an account to use their tools. The greatest challenge of this page is the vast amount of information – it's scattered everywhere and can be hard to wrap your mind around it. The goal of this book is to organize and streamline the information and make it more useable in real life situations.

The tools that I have found most helpful on the TRICARE website are:

- **The Plan Finder Tool.** At the top of the TRICARE page, click "Plans & Eligibility." Through a series of questions, this tool will identify the TRICARE plans available to you and your family. Click the "Compare Plans" option to view plans side-by-side (works best on a computer, not a phone). Chapter 3 of this book walks you through different scenarios of the Plan Finder Tool.

- **The What's Covered Tool.** At the top of the TRICARE page, click "What's Covered." You can search by keyword or browse by category to see what is covered or excluded. See Chapter 4 and our YouTube channel at **www.youtube.com/@thetricareguy** for tips on your benefits through this tool. The tool can yield some misleading results which we will help you navigate.

- **The Cost Tool.** This was one of my favorite tools that allowed you to compare the cost of different plans by just clicking a few buttons. It worked great, but sadly the Cost Compare Tool was retired in January 2025 and replaced by a less-flexible display of costs, organized by plan and sponsor status. The data is accurate, but not as elegant as the previous tool. Please see Chapter 6 for a more detailed discussion of finding Cost information on the TRICARE website.

For the sake of completeness, I will mention there is a fourth tool called "Find a Provider." Regrettably, that one falls short for a number of reasons. Please review Chapter 5 to understand this tool, its shortfalls, and strategies for finding TRICARE providers. By mastering the suite of TRICARE online tools, you will be able to find answers for the most common questions about your benefits.

Regional Contractor Web Portals

Web portals of the regional contractors (East, West, and Overseas) are where you will create log-in accounts for you and your family members to file claims, upload documents, set up direct deposit, message your regional contractor, manage enrollment, and more. See Appendix A for more information about these portals.

Explore your portal. Create an account and look around. You may create accounts in one, two, or all three regional portals; this will not affect your enrollment or benefits. Anyone planning to travel internationally should create an account on the TRICARE Overseas portal before leaving the States. Each portal has different features, so the best way to learn is by exploring. As you browse the portal, your understanding and confidence will increase.

Expert tip: If you anticipate international travel, create an online account in the TRICARE Overseas web portal for yourself and all adult members of your family. All care outside the United States is managed by TRICARE Overseas, so having an account pre-made will expedite things if you find yourself hospitalized. The site's anti-fraud measures make creation of a new account difficult or completely impossible when outside the U.S.

Expert tip: Before moving or traveling overseas, install one or more calling apps on your phone such as Google Voice, Vonage, or Zoom Phone. Create an account and make some practice calls. This allows you to do two things:

- First, it allows you to call American toll-free numbers from overseas at no cost. Without such an app, it might be impossible to call toll-free numbers from abroad.

- Second, if you need assistance, you can call the TRICARE regional offices, like Singapore and UK. With calling apps, this costs just a penny or two per minute. It is vastly more expensive if using cell phone calling. You can even use the app to call local numbers in the country that you are visiting without having a SIM card for that country.

MyCare Overseas™ Mobile App

International SOS, the contractor that manages TRICARE Overseas, offers the MyCare Overseas™ app to access health information for international users. You can find and install it via your app store but be careful! There is another International SOS app intended for ISOS corporate (non-military) customers. Be sure to get the right app! You can access the web app at **top.internationalsos.com/beneficiary**

The MyCare Overseas™ app allows you to:
- View your appointments and referrals
- Track your overseas claims

The Ultimate Guide to TRICARE

- Locate in-network providers
- Find country information, including emergency phone numbers, cultural tips, and medical risks
- Get translation assistance for medical care, when necessary.

The app is most useful for those enrolled in TRICARE Overseas Prime, meaning active duty members and their families since retirees cannot enroll in Prime Overseas. It has lesser functionality for all others, such as retirees enrolled in Select Overseas. To use the app, you must create a new ID and password, different from your account on the TRICARE Overseas web portal.

Official TRICARE Social Media

TRICARE and MHS are present on social media. The official TRICARE Facebook page serves as a conduit to push information to the community about military health benefits. It isn't a good way to ask questions about your specific needs. If you post a question, they normally will just say, "Give us a call." We do recommend that you follow their page to receive TRICARE news and events in your Facebook feed.

Official TRICARE social media accounts include:
- Facebook: **www.facebook.com/TRICARE**
- X/Twitter: **@Tricare**
- YouTube channel: **www.youtube.com/Tricare**
- LinkedIn: Search for **"Defense Health Agency"** or **"Military Health System."**

TRICARE Guy Social Media

The TRICARE Guy – the author of this book – is also active on social media. You will find our groups to be welcoming and collaborative. Our #1 rule is courtesy and respect, so it is a very supportive community. Our social media groups include:

- **TRICARE® Around the World**
  www.facebook.com/groups/tricareatw
- **TRICARE® in Thailand**
  www.facebook.com/groups/TricareInThailand
- **TRICARE® in Germany**
  www.facebook.com/groups/TricareInGermany
- **TRICARE® in the Philippines**
  www.facebook.com/groups/TricareInPhilippines
- **TRICARE® for New Moms and Moms-to-be**
  www.facebook.com/groups/tricare4moms
- **The TRICARE Guy YouTube channel**
  www.youtube.com/@thetricareguy

In these groups, you can interact with the author as well as thousands of TRICARE users around the world. No matter where you find yourself, you are likely to find others nearby for current, local information. We also have a number of subject matter experts who can dive deep into your benefit questions.

MHS Nurse Advice Line

One of the greatest resources for TRICARE beneficiaries is the MHS Nurse Advice Line, available 24/7/365. Staffed by registered nurses, this call center can help you with questions about your benefits and, unlike your regional contractor, can offer medical guidance based on your specific symptoms. Contact the MHS Nurse Advice Line to:

- Obtain recommendations for the most appropriate care.
- Speak to a pediatric nurse for concerns about your child.
- Find an urgent care or emergency care facility near you.
- Schedule same or next day appointments if enrolled in a military hospital or clinic.
- Get an online "absence excuse" or "sick slip" for ADSM, subject to service or command requirements.

The Advice Line is open around the clock, so you can connect at any time by phone, video chat, or text chat via their portal at **mhsnurseadviceline.com**

Expert tip: You can launch a chat session without logging in, but we recommend that you log in first for two reasons:

- If logged in, you can download a transcript of the chat session. This is useful for reviewing talking points.

- Logging in first speeds up the verification of your identity and it authorizes you to discuss family members linked to your TRICARE account. If you don't log in, there is a lengthy verification process at the start of the call.

The following is a complete listing of country-specific numbers for the MHS Nurse Advice Line. The website says they provide services only to beneficiaries in these specific countries or regions, but we have successfully used their services even when not in one of these locations. It's worth a try, when you have the need.

United States, Guam, Puerto Rico, Cuba, Diego Garcia: 1-800-TRICARE (874-2273)

Bahrain: 800-06432

Belgium: 0800-81933

Germany: 0800-071-3516

Greece: 00-800-4414-1013

Italy: 800-979721

Japan: Landline: 888-901-7144;
Mobile: 0066-33-821820 or 0120-996-985

South Korea: 888-901-7144; mobile: 080-500-4011

Spain: 900-82-2740

Turkey: 00-800-44-882-5287

United Kingdom: 0800-028-3263

Universal International Freephone (from participating European nations): 00-800-4759-2330

Case Management

If you're being treated for chronic, high-risk, high-cost, catastrophic or terminal illness, you can get case management services at no cost to you. Case managers are usually nurses or social workers experienced in helping patients and families navigate complex health care and support systems.

To locate a case manager, contact:

- Your regional contractor
- Your military hospital or clinic
- A Beneficiary Counseling and Assistance Coordinator (see next section).

Benefit and Debt Counseling

TRICARE beneficiaries have access to specialized counseling for benefits and debts related to unpaid TRICARE bills.

- **Beneficiary Counseling and Assistance Coordinators** (BCAC) educate beneficiaries and help with questions related to TRICARE eligibility, enrollment, referrals/authorizations, and issues with claims processing.

- **Debt Collection Assistance Officers** (DCAO) assist with debt collection due to unpaid TRICARE claims. The debt must be in collections or listed on your credit report.

To search for a BCAC or DCAO by state or country, visit **tricare.mil/bcacdcao**. Each of these resources should be used only <u>after</u> you have tried to resolve the matter through your regional contractor.

Adult Children with Disabilities

As explained in Chapter 2, a severely disabled adult child can remain on TRICARE throughout their lifetime. Your adult child can remain on Prime or Select until they become eligible for Medicare, at which time they will switch to TRICARE for Life (TFL). Coverage can continue even after the death of both parents, but you must plan carefully for their ongoing care.

The following tips are compiled from members in our Facebook group "TRICARE Around the World." This is an informal list, but it is useful from those who have been in your shoes. It should serve as a springboard for further research.

- Use ECHO benefits as much as possible before retirement. Retiree families cannot use ECHO.

- Your child may enroll in Prime or Select. The farther away from an MTF they are, the harder it becomes to use Prime.

- Your disabled child may be eligible for Medicaid and Social Security benefits.

- Survivor Benefit Plan (SBP) may be assigned to the child rather than spouse, giving the child lifetime cash benefits. It might be best to set up a special needs trust and assign the benefits to the trust. Consult an estate lawyer who specializes in military benefits.

- Set up an accounting system to track expenses for food, housing, etc. You will need to demonstrate the full living expenses of your child. This requirement continues even after the death of the parents, so you will need a solid guardianship plan to take care of these details.

- Ensure the child's military ID card is renewed before each expiration. If the card expires, it can be a major chore to re-establish the ID.

MHS Genesis Patient Portal

The MHS Genesis Patient Portal is an online resource to access patient records and manage care through the Military Health System. This system completed global rollout in 2024, and replaced the previous portal, TRICARE Online (TOL). Not all files and records from TOL ported over to Genesis, so you might find items missing from your medical history.

MHS Genesis works best for those on Prime, who get care mostly within an MTF. You can use this system to:

- Book appointments
- Securely message your health care team
- Request prescription refills
- View and download health data and lab results

Learn more about this vital resource including how to create an account at **tricare.mil/mhsgenesis**

988 Crisis Hotline

In 2020, the U.S. Department of Health and Human Services, together with the VA, launched the 988 nationwide crisis hotline. This three-digit number links together more than 200 existing state & local call centers, including suicide and crisis care for veterans. Most of the older 10-digit crisis line phone numbers still work, but calling or texting is a quick and easy way to connect with local, confidential care 24/7. Press 1 after calling to connect with counselors trained in the needs and resources of veterans.

From their website at **988lifeline.org**, there are options to initiate a web-based chat session, or a video session for using American Sign Language (ASL). Resources also are available for loved ones of veterans in crisis, to advise ways that family and friends may help in times of need. If you (or someone you know) are in need of urgent care, please use this valuable resource.

TRICARE Service Centers (TSC)

TRICARE Service Centers in overseas locations are available for in-person assistance to TRICARE beneficiaries. These are found at some military bases around the world. The TSC can assist with care in a military clinic or hospital, care with a foreign provider off base, and answer questions about eligibility, enrollment, claims processing, and more.

TSCs can be found in:

- **Eurasia/Middle East:** Bahrain, Brussels, Germany, Greece, Italy, Spain, Turkey, and the United Kingdom
- **The Americas:** Guantanamo Bay and Puerto Rico
- **Pacific:** Japan, Korea, Guam

To find specific TSC locations and contact information, visit **www.tricare.mil/tsc**.

Retired Activities Offices (RAO)

Retired Activities Offices (RAO) are often affiliated with U.S. embassies, consulates, or military bases and provide a great number of services for the local retiree community. RAOs are staffed by trained volunteers who aid and assist retired military members, their spouses, and surviving family members. In some countries, RAOs can receive U.S. mail for retirees in the area through cooperation with APO/FPO services. To find one near you, call the nearest U.S. embassy or consulate, or ask within your local community.

In the Philippines, RAOs play a very robust role in helping vets to access to the VA clinic in Manila and offering mail forwarding service to retirees living in the country. This can include receipt of prescriptions sent from Express Scripts home delivery. Learn more about this valuable service in Chapter 9.

Veterans Service Offices (VSO)

Across the USA and in many locations around the world, you will find trained volunteers at Veterans Service Offices (VSO) who are committed to serving veterans, their families, and survivors of deceased service members.

VSOs will assist with a great many needs, including helping members apply for benefits or decedent affairs after a veteran passes away. They can help the surviving spouse apply for Social Security, VA benefits, Medicare, TRICARE, and more. Examples of VSOs include Veterans of Foreign Wars (VFW), American Legion, Disabled American Veterans (DAV), and many others.

One way to find a nearby VSO is to ask within the military community in your local area. You probably know someone who is a member of a local chapter. You also can search Facebook or the internet for local organizations. The VA maintains a list of Veterans Service Organizations at **www.va.gov/VSO/**

VA Assistance Overseas

The VA provides Overseas Military Services Coordinators (OMSC) in select overseas locations to assist service members approaching separation and U.S. veterans living or working overseas. The OMSC are located primarily near major military bases in select countries around the world. OMSCs will also advise the dependents or eligible family members of veterans.

As of this writing, OMSC advisors are located in Germany, Italy, Japan, and the UK. They can be accessed remotely for those living in other countries. To locate an advisor near you, visit **www.benefits.va.gov/benefits/oms_Coordinators.asp**

More information about VA resources can be found in Chapter 9 (for the Philippines) and Chapter 10 for all international locations.

Global Resources

Official TRICARE website: www.tricare.mil

Military hospitals and clinics worldwide:
www.tricare.mil/Military-Hospitals-and-Clinics

MHS Nurse Advice Line: www.mhsnurseadviceline.com

Contact Wizard: tricare.mil/ContactUs/CallUs

This is an online tool to guide you to the right phone number or address for your needs.

TRICARE East
Humana Military: **www.tricare-east.com**

TRICARE West
TriWest: **tricare-bene.triwest.com**

TRICARE Overseas
International SOS: **www.tricare-overseas.com**

TRICARE For Life (TFL)
Wisconsin Physician Services: **www.tricare4u.com**

U.S. Family Health Plan: www.usfhp.com

Active Duty Dental Program (ADDP)/TRICARE Dental Program (TDP)
United Concordia: **secure.addp-ucci.com**

TRICARE Overseas Regional Call Centers
(open 24 hours, Monday - Friday local time)

Europe, Middle East & Africa:
44-20-8762-8384 from overseas
1-877-678-1207 from a U.S. phone

Latin American and Canada:
1-215-942-8393 from overseas
1-877-451-8659 from a U.S. phone

Puerto Rico: 1-877-867-1091

Asia-Pacific:
65-6339-2676 from overseas
1-877-678-1208 from a U.S. phone

Australia/Oceana:
61-2-9273-2710 from overseas
1-877-678-1209 from a U.S. phone

Appendix A:
Regional Web Portals

THE FOLLOWING IS AN OVERVIEW of the web portals of the three Regional Contractors: TRICARE East, TRICARE West, and TRICARE Overseas. This appendix will help explain the key features of your web portal.

Overview

Web addresses of the regional portals are:

- **East:** www.tricare-east.com
- **West:** tricare-bene.triwest.com
- **Overseas:** www.tricare-overseas.com

Each portal is different; you will have to get accustomed to the layout of your particular one and where to find each feature. Create an account in your region's portal and just start exploring. The web sites are highly subject to change, so any descriptions offered in this Appendix may be superseded at any time.

- If your family is geographically separated, you may need to use more than one regional portal.

- You can have accounts for one, two, or all three portals. Creating these accounts will not change your enrollment or benefits.

- It is exceedingly difficult to create an account for TRICARE Overseas when you are outside the United States, due to strict anti-fraud measures that are used. If you anticipate international travel, you are <u>strongly</u> urged to create an account in the TRICARE Overseas web portal

<u>before</u> leaving the United States. This can vastly expedite care if you are hospitalized overseas.

Creating Family Member Accounts

Before any family member can create an online account, they must be enrolled in DEERS (the Defense Enrollment Eligibility Reporting System), which establishes their eligibility for TRICARE benefits. Contact the DEERS/ID card office at any military base for assistance or visit the MilConnect site at **milconnect.dmdc.osd.mil/**

Each authorized family member should have their own account in their regional portal. You may have to call to set up accounts for younger children due to privacy rules. If you are enrolled in TRICARE East or West but want to file a claim for care received overseas, you should create an online account on the TRICARE Overseas site. You can have accounts on multiple regional portals simultaneously.

There are two ways to create an account: Either with a dedicated ID and password or with a DoD Self-Service (DS) Logon. The DS account can be used across a broad range of DoD sites. The method that you choose may depend on:

- Whether or not you have a Common Access Card (CAC).
- Whether or not you live in the United States.

If you have a CAC, then you may already have a DS Logon. If you do not have a CAC and are living outside the United States, then creating a DS Logon may be difficult or impossible. In that case, create a portal account with a dedicated login name and password. Each contractor portal provides instructions for creating your account. The portals are linked to DEERS to instantly validate eligibility. The TRICARE Overseas portal is tied to the email address you listed in DEERS, so first make sure that your information in DEERS is current.

Linking Family Member Accounts

Once each family member has their own online account, they can be linked. Linking accounts does two important things:

- It allows you, from your own account, to submit and manage claims for all family members.
- It signifies consent for you to speak with TRICARE representatives about the medical needs of adult family members.

Even if your account is linked to a family member, some claims will remain confidential due to their sensitive nature. This confidentiality can start as young as age 13. Sensitive claims will not be viewable from the linked account of a family member. Examples of such claims include:

- Abortion
- Alcoholism
- Drug abuse
- Pregnancy
- Venereal Disease
- Sexually Transmitted Disease
- AIDS/HIV
- Sexual assault
- Domestic violence

When a minor child turns 18, all parental access to their account ends. The link can be re-established after their 18th birthday but only with your child's consent.

Establishing Direct Deposit

We strongly encourage you to set up direct deposit for all family members, particularly if you live or travel overseas. **TRICARE direct deposit reimbursements can go only to U.S. banks.** If you do not set up direct deposit, a paper check will be mailed to you. **For most banks, you must physically**

be in the United States to open an account, so make sure that you have a U.S. checking account <u>before</u> moving overseas.

Search for "Direct Deposit" in your portal's menu. This will bring up a list of all family members. Starting with the sponsor, enter all the required banking information. You will be able to reuse the same banking information for your linked family members if you want deposits to go to the same bank account. **For minor children, direct deposit authorization will expire on their 18th birthday.** They will have to re-establish their direct deposit preferences after turning 18.

Expert tip: If the Direct Deposit form has both a start date and an end date, do NOT leave the end date blank. Members of our Facebook group have found that if the end date is blank, it will end immediately. This has caused weeks of frustration for some of our members. Choose an end date as far into the future as you like, and then the set-up will "stick."

Claim Status

Contractor portals have rudimentary tracking capabilities for your claims. In the TRICARE Overseas portal, you will receive instant notification in the message center when you file your claim online. If you submit your claim by fax or mail, you may not receive confirmation until the claim is fully processed and approved or denied. This can take two months.

If you want the current status of your claim, it is always best to call. Response to written messages is slow, and frequently their written answers are not particularly helpful. There is a particular "gotcha" in the system – once you send a written inquiry about a claim, they have 30 days to respond. If you call during those 30 days, they will say: *"We are working on your written request; we cannot give status over the phone."* So, skip the written message and just call them.

When processing is complete, you will receive an Explanation of Benefits (EOB) which provides a breakdown of the allowable costs, your copay/cost-share, covered amounts, and how much counts towards your deductible and annual catastrophic cap. EOBs may either be on a claim-by-claim basis or they may bundle multiple claims into a monthly EOB. If you ever have a billing issue with a provider, always wait until you have your EOB to see how much TRICARE says you owe.

Message Center

The Message Center provides a secure way to communicate with your Regional Contractor. If needed, you can send your documents through the Message Center to support a claim. Make sure to include the claim number in the subject line and written on the documents so that they can be attached to the appropriate claim.

TRICARE Overseas generally takes two to four weeks to answer questions sent through the Message Center, but their responses are often vague and unresponsive to the actual question that was asked. If you call within 30 days after submitting a written inquiry, they may decline to answer your question by phone because they have 30 days to respond to your written request. For this reason, I almost never message them with a question; I just call and get my answer over the phone.

Appendix B:
Acronyms

ABA – Applied Behavioral Analysis

ACA – Affordable Care Act

ACN – Autism Care Navigator

ACD – Autism Care Demonstration

ACS – American Citizen Services

ADDP – Active Duty Dental Program

ADFM – Active Duty Family Member

ADSM – Active Duty Service Member

APO/FPO – Army Post Office/Fleet Post Office

BCAC – Beneficiary Counseling and Assistance Coordinator

CAC – Common Access Card

CDC – Centers for Disease Control and Prevention

CHAMPUS – Civilian Health and Medical Program of the Uniformed Services

CHCBP – Continued Health Care Benefit Program

CHAMPVA – Civilian Health and Medical Program of the Department of Veterans Affairs

CMAC – CHAMPUS Maximum Allowable Charge

CONUS – Continental United States

CPAP – Continuous Positive Airway Pressure

CPT – Current Professional Terminology

CRBA – Consular Report of Birth Abroad

DAV – Disabled American Veterans

DBN – DoD Benefit Number

DCAO – Debt Collection Assistance Officer

DCO – Direct Care Only

DEERS – Defense Enrollment Eligibility Reporting System

DHS – Defense Health Agency

DME – Durable Medical Equipment

DoD – Department of Defense

DPP – Deployment Prescription Program

DVA – Department of Veterans Affairs

ECHO – Extended Care Health Option

EFMP – Exceptional Family Member Program

EOB – Explanation of Benefits

ETP – Exception to Policy

FDA – U.S. Food and Drug Administration

FEDVIP – Federal Employees Dental and Vision Insurance Program

FEHB – Federal Employees Health Benefits

FHP – Family Health Plan

FMP – Foreign Medical Program

HIPAA – Health Insurance Portability and Accountability Act

HP&DP – Health Promotion and Disease Prevention

ICD – International Classification of Disease

ISOS – International SOS

JUSMAG – Joint U.S. Military Advisory Group

MHS – Military Health System

MoH – Medal of Honor

MTF – Military Treatment Facility

NOAA – National Oceanic and Atmospheric Administration

NORA – Naval Ophthalmic Readiness Activity

OHI – Other Health Insurance

OMSC – Overseas Military Services Coordinator

OSA – Obstructive Sleep Apnea

OTC – Over the Counter (drugs)

P&T – Permanent & Total Disability (VA classification)

PCM – Primary Care Manager

PLDT – Philippine Long-Distance Telephone

POS – Point of Service

PSA – Prime Service Area

QLE – Qualifying Life Event

RACHAP – Retiree-At-Cost Hearing Aid Program

RHAPP – Retiree Hearing Aid Purchase Program

RAO – Retired Activities Office

SCD – Service-Connected Disability

SEP – Special Enrollment Period

SOFA – Status of Forces Agreement

SSA – Social Security Administration

SSDI – Social Security Disability Insurance

SSN – Social Security Number

TAMP – Transitional Assistance Management Program

TDP – TRICARE Dental Program

TFL – TRICARE for Life

TOP – TRICARE Overseas Program

TRR – TRICARE Retired Reserve

TRS – TRICARE Reserve Select

TSC – TRICARE Service Center

TYA – TRICARE Young Adult

TYA-S – TRICARE Young Adult-Select

TYA-P – TRICARE Young Adult-Prime

USFHP – U.S. Family Health Plan

USPHS – U.S. Public Health Service

USMTF – United States Military Treatment Facility

VA – (Department of) Veterans Affairs

VADIP – VA Dental Insurance Plan

VFW – Veterans of Foreign Wars

VSI – Voluntary Separation Incentive

VSO – Veterans Service Organizations

WPS – Wisconsin Physician Service

Appendix C:
Age-Related TRICARE Events

THE FOLLOWING ARE TRICARE EVENTS based on age. Details can be found in the listed references.

Age 0 (newborn): Auto-enrolled in TRICARE Prime, Prime Remote or Select based on location and status of parents. **Reference: Chapter 2, "Newborns"**

Age 90 days (stateside) or 120 days (overseas): Deadline for DEERS enrollment for continuous coverage under TRICARE. **Reference: Chapter 2, "Newborns"**

Age 6: Cut-off for well-child care, which is a special slate of exams and assessments. **NOTE**: This benefit ends the day before the child's sixth birthday. **Reference: www.tricare.mil/CoveredServices/IsItCovered/WellChildCare**

Age 21, Cut-off for children's coverage under sponsor's plan if not enrolled in a qualifying institution of higher learning. **Reference: Chapter 2, "Adult Children"**

Age 21: Deadline to certify adult children with significant disabilities to remain on parent's TRICARE plan. **Reference: Chapter 2, "Adult Children with Disabilities"**

Age 23: Cut-off for children's coverage under sponsor's plan if enrolled full-time in a qualifying institute of higher learning. **Reference: Chapter 2, "Adult Children"**

Age 26: Cut-off for coverage under TRICARE Young Adult. **Reference: Chapter 7 "TRICARE Young Adult"**

Age 60: Transition from TRICARE Retired Reserve to TRICARE Prime or Select for gray area retirees and their dependents. **Reference: Chapter 7 "TRICARE Retired Reserve"**

Age 62: The earliest age that retirees can begin age-based Social Security benefits. This is not a TRICARE event, but people often confuse this age with the start date of Medicare, which is 65.
Reference: Chapter 8, "Medicare & TRICARE for Life"

30-day window <u>before</u> age 65: The timeframe during which a retired sponsor can get their INDEF ID card.
Reference: Chapter 8, "Updating Your Military ID Card

Age 65: Enrollment in Medicare and transition to TRICARE for Life for all TRICARE beneficiaries. Exceptions apply for ADSM and ADFM and certain working adults. If one is drawing Social Security by age 65, then their Medicare enrollment is automatic, and fees will be drawn from Social Security starting at 65. If not, they will have to make other payment arrangements for Medicare until their Social Security benefits begin.
Reference: Chapter 8, "Medicare & TRICARE for Life"

Age-Based Medical Benefits: There are other age-based determinants for medical benefits such as mammography, colonoscopy, and certain vaccines. We are not listing them here because they are subject to change based on evolving medical guidance and can be affected by an individual's medical history. Work closely with your doctor to determine when certain age-based health assessments are appropriate and covered.

Appendix D:
TRICARE Claim Checklist

THIS IS YOUR "ONE-STOP CHECKLIST" for filing your claims with TRICARE. Official guidance is scattered far and wide, with tips from Tricare.mil, TRICARE Overseas (ISOS), the TRICARE claim form (DD-2642), and various other websites. We have done the legwork to draw it all together in one spot and include valuable practical tips gained from personal experience.

Carefully following these steps will avoid 99% of the reasons that claims are commonly denied. Do not take shortcuts or work from memory! Read this checklist every time. If you do this, you can expect most claims to be approved in just a few weeks.

1. **Follow TRICARE's own filing tips. _Reference_:** tricare.mil/PatientResources/Claims/MedicalClaims/FilingTips

   a. **Keep DEERS current for all family members**, especially after an address change or changes in your family. Any incorrect information in DEERS can cause your claim to be delayed or denied.

   b. **Use form DD-2642 to file your claim.** The form can be downloaded from **tricare.mil** or from your regional contractor's website.

   c. **Fill in all boxes fully and accurately.**

   d. **List the diagnosis code in Block 8a.** If unknown, state a full description of the reason for care in Block 8a.

   e. **Sign the form!** Claims submitted without a signature will be denied payment. For some reason, the signature block often prints with a big X through it. This seems to be dependent on the software on your computer; the form will be fine for some people yet lined out for others. You must manually remove the X.

f. **If you were injured at work or by another party, include DD Form 2527** (Statement of Personal Injury). See Chapter 13, "Third Party Liability" for more details.

g. **File claims with Other Health Insurance (OHI) first.** You must include the OHI explanation of benefits (EOB) when you submit your TRICARE claim. **Failing to settle OHI first constitutes insurance fraud and is subject to prosecution!**

h. **Keep copies of <u>everything</u>.** Documents can and do get lost during filing.

i. **Send claims to the right address.** One processor will not forward to another if you send it to the wrong one. See the section in Chapter 13: "Who Do You File With?"

j. **File on time.** You have one year to file for care received in the States; three years for care received overseas.

k. **Submit each claim separately.** Bundling multiple claims is likely to cause confusion.

l. **Pat yourself on the back for a job well done.**

2. **File with the correct agency.**

a. **If you are enrolled with TRICARE Overseas,** file with TRICARE Overseas even if you get care in the U.S. *Reference:* http://www.tricare-overseas.com/ beneficiaries/resources/traveling-beneficiaries

b. **If you are enrolled in a stateside TRICARE plan and get medical care overseas**, file with TRICARE Overseas (not with your U.S. regional contractor). This is true for all TRICARE beneficiaries. *Reference:* https://www.tricare.mil/traveling

c. **If you are enrolled in a stateside plan and get medical care in a different region** (for example, you are in TRICARE East but get care in the West region), file with your home regional contractor.

3. **Digital format for online claims:**

- **Scan in grayscale or black & white, not color.** The TOP claim processing system is incapable of handling color attachments. Research your scanner's instructions to learn how to do this; each is different. **Even a black & white document should not be scanned in color** because the resulting file format is different than a grayscale scan.
  Reference: Pop-up window in the TOP claims portal.

- **When submitting electronically, put all of the documents into a single multi-page file.** While the portal allows upload of multiple attachments, they warn you not to do so. On a Mac, you can combine documents into a single PDF file using the Preview app. On a Windows computer, you may need third-party software to combine documents, or you can paste multiple documents into a Word file.

- **File size should not exceed 8 MB.**

4. **Block 8A is your friend!** Use Block 8A on form DD-2642 to explain the reason for care. If it is not clear why treatment was needed, the claim may be rejected. If you cannot fit full details in Block 8A, write: "See attached page" then include details on a separate sheet. Do not assume the reviewer knows anything of your prior history; make it easy for them to understand.

5. **Annotate/Mark Up Your Documents**

a. At the top of your claim form, write **"Beneficiary Paid Provider Directly"** and **the amount paid** to clarify that TRICARE should reimburse you, not the hospital.
   Reference: www.tricare.mil/proofofpayment

At the top of all other pages, write the patient's name and the sponsor's SSN or DBN.
Reference: "Reminders" at bottom of DD-2642 page 1.

c. **Block 13 (Payment):** Indicate if you want to be paid in U.S. dollars or foreign currency (e.g., Euros, pesos, baht, yen, etc.) Not all currencies are available, so call ISOS if you have questions. For Proof of Payment, check "Yes" if you paid all or part of the bill directly to the provider.

6. **Document translation is optional.** ISOS will accept documents in a foreign language but paperwork in English might be processed faster. Ensure that the patient's name is written using English (Latin) characters, not transliterated into a foreign alphabet. Your name in Cyrillic or katakana is bound to cause problems.

7. **Pay with plastic.** Paying medical bills with cash can be a red flag for fraud, especially in the Philippines. If you do pay with cash, be prepared for greater scrutiny. Include ATM or bank receipts with your claim for the cash withdrawal. If possible, pay with a credit card or debit card to avoid this complication. See our discussion in Chapter 9 entitled "Pay with Plastic."

8. **The most important step of all!** After submitting your claim, **wait 24 hours/one business day then call** to ensure that it was correctly received. The questions to ask when you call:

a. **Was my claim received?**

b. **What pages do you see?** *(Have your copies ready so that you can compare.)*

c. **Are all the pages legible?** *(Sometimes the pages get garbled in transmission.)*

d. **Do you see any problems?** *(The representative should check the entire claim for obvious errors or problems. This is not a guarantee of approval, but it can head off problems early in the process.)*

e. **Confirm that the reimbursement will come to <u>you</u>, not to the provider, if you paid the provider directly.**

We have found the service representatives to be quite helpful during these reviews. If they tell you that an attachment is garbled or missing, you do not have to re-submit the entire claim. Create a message in the Message Center with the subject "General Question", write the Claim Number in the body of your message, and attach the file. Annotate claim number on the top of the page you are sending. The new file should be added automatically to your existing claim. Call back the next business day to double-check.

9. **Seek assistance.** There are many resources available to assist with your claim. This includes customer representatives at the **TRICARE Overseas regional offices**. They are available by phone 24 hours, Monday through Friday, in their local time zone, so that you do not have to call in the middle of the night.

At major military bases around the world, you will find **TRICARE Service Centers (TSC)** to assist with questions and claims. They are also knowledgeable about health care options off base, which can be helpful to those on Select who do not have a PCM to give referrals. **Retired Activities Offices (RAO)** worldwide can help or will refer you to appropriate resources. **VFW posts and other veterans' groups** often have subject matter experts to help. See Chapter 14 for contact information.

10. **Join our Facebook group *"TRICARE Around the World"*** to connect with thousands of military members, retirees, families, and caregivers worldwide. You will be able to interact with the author and other experts. We are committed to providing fast, reliable information to all who ask. We also host other groups including **TRICARE in Thailand, Germany, and the Philippines**, plus **TRICARE for new moms and moms-to-be.**

Stay Involved!

Through the *TRICARE Around the World* community, we are trying to make life better for our military family. Here are some things you can do to help:

- PLEASE leave **a 5-star review** where you bought this book. A paragraph or two from you helps lifts in the search results, allowing us to reach even more of the military community.

- **Visit www.theTRICAREguy.com to join our mailing list.** Send us your ideas on how to make future editions of this book even better. We welcome your input. This edition addresses a broad range of feedback from readers like you.

- **Donate a book!** Buy additional copies to donate to local veterans groups, VSOs, RAOs, VA hospital, local library (on base or off base). As an alternative, ask your librarian to order this book to help other military families.

- **Join our global community.** Our Facebook group is not just a place to ask questions, but also to share with others what you have learned about your TRICARE benefits. Our community needs you!

See you online and on your global travels!

www.theTRICAREguy.com

About the Author

John D. Letaw is a retired Naval officer who served on six different ships in the Pacific fleet throughout his career. Later, as a defense contractor, he helped to develop and deploy tactical software to ensure mission success for Joint forces. From 2009-2012, John served as the Asia-Pacific Regional Manager of the Transition Assistance Program (TAP) in Iwakuni, Japan, teaching classes in career transition and counseling military members and their spouses about life after the military. During that time, John and his wife Pen also ran a youth program at the station chapel.

In retirement, John turned his attention to TRICARE and how to make it accessible to all. This effort sprang from his family's international lifestyle, which gave them deep insight into using TRICARE health benefits in a variety of settings – from remote mountain villages in Japan to gleaming 5-star hospitals in Bangkok, as a SOFA-status contractor overseas, and as a retiree in Hawaii on Medicare.

John's Facebook group, ***TRICARE Around the World***, is the world's largest and most active online community dedicated to sharing information about TRICARE. With 25,000 members and growing, the questions, stories, challenges and victories shared by group members have had a profound influence on the development of this book.

For links to our community or to sign up for our newsletter, visit the author's website at www.TheTricareGuy.com

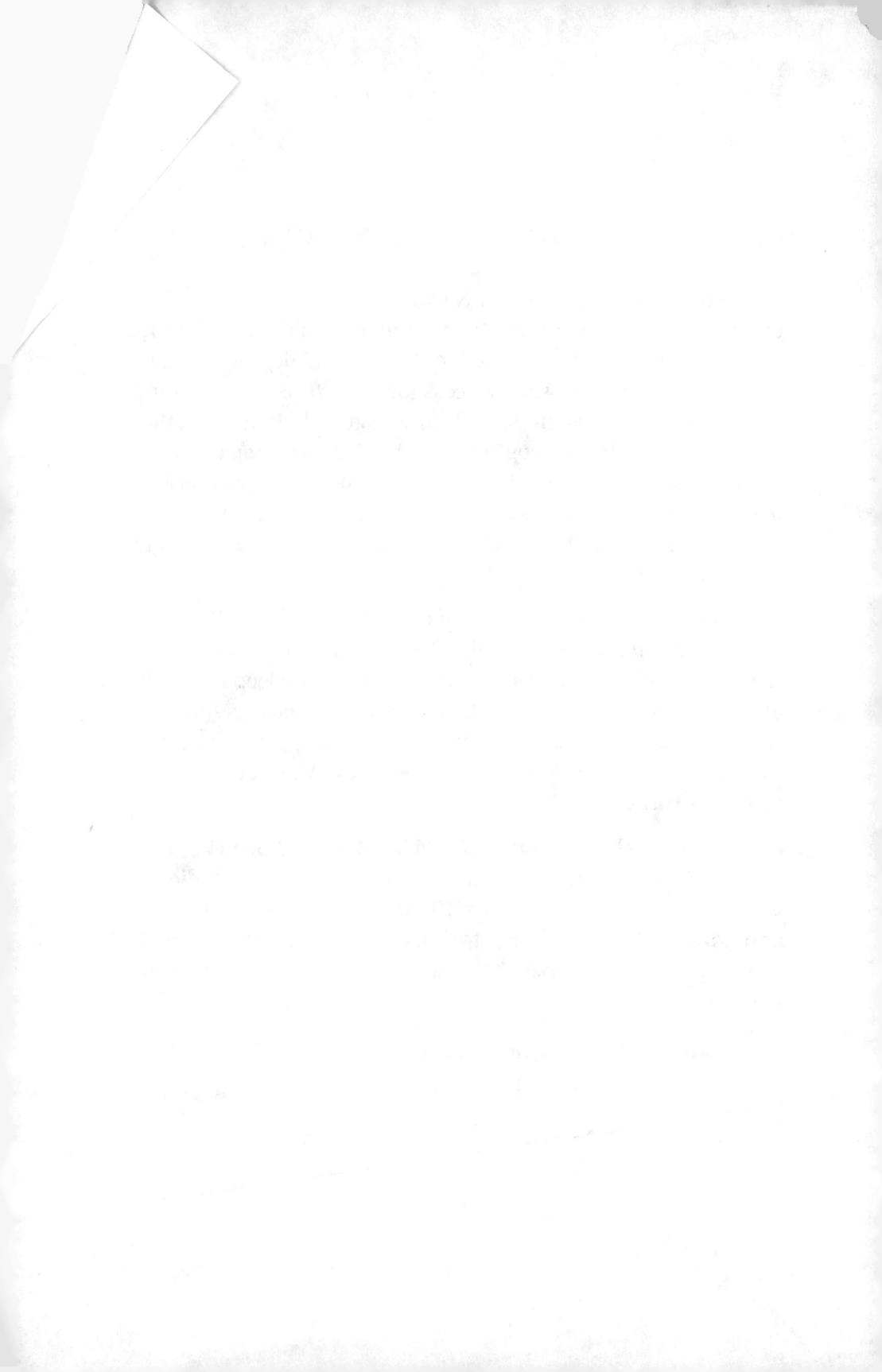